Foreword

In recent years there has developed among physical therapists a growing interest in the theory and practice of manipulative therapy. This is especially apparent upon reviewing the current journals of the physical therapy associations of Canada, Great Britain, America, and Australia. Within the last decade manipulation has become accepted much more readily both by physicians and therapists, as part of the therapists' field of expertise. Courses at both graduate and undergraduate levels are now being offered in manipulation, their objective being to reach and teach the physical therapy populace. These courses are offered by therapists for therapists. Unfortunately, along with this growth in scope of practice, new literature, especially in the form of books, has not materialized. By far the greater number of books presently available are written by physicians, and they are aimed principally at the physicians. The books by Maitland of Australia are an obvious exception. Although these are a very valuable asset to all therapists currently practicing manipulative therapy, they often do not fulfill the need, as expressed by therapists, for an introductory text on spinal manipulation. Mr. Nwuga's text, *Manipulation of the Spine* therefore comes at a very opportune time.

Within his text Mr. Nwuga has put great emphasis on the physical examination and assessment of the patient. With this I concur. Mr. Nwuga, not being a physician, has quite rightly omitted long sections on pathology and theories of joint dysfunction. Instead, he has placed the emphasis on the areas of his own expertise. No particular "school of thought" has been expounded in preference of others. Mr. Nwuga has presented a comprehensive, introductory text, explaining how different therapy techniques may be utilized in different circumstances. Being a therapist myself and one involved in teaching and practicing manipulative therapy, I agree with Mr. Nwuga's format.

On reading the text one realizes the extent of Mr. Nwuga's experience in this field. He shares this experience and knowledge with his readers in the section on case presentations. For one not too familiar with the practice of manipulation this should prove to be a valuable asset. One can then move logically from the sections on assessment and examination, to treatment, and finally see how the author himself tackled specific problems.

I hope this book will find a place on the shelves of all therapists interested in spinal manipulation. To such readers and Mr. Vince Nwuga I express my sincere good wishes.

R. P. Walmsley, M.Sc., M.C.S.P.,
Associate Professor and Head,
Physical Therapy Program,
School of Rehabilitation Therapy,
Queen's University,
Kingston, Ontario,
Canada.

Preface

This book discusses an old therapeutic modality which is gaining a heartening recognition again after languishing in the doldrums of neglect for quite a while.

Although the book is directed primarily at the Physical Therapist, both undergraduate and graduate, it is hoped that all practitioners involved with manual therapy, whatever ideological stripe they are wearing, or whichever school of thought they subscribe to, will find something of value as they thumb through its pages. It is also meant for those people who share my wish to make a contribution toward the dissemination of knowledge and the teaching of skills which will help to mollify or extirpate the agonies attendant on the ubiquitous back pain.

The techniques of manipulation I have discussed are related to the vertebral column and the pelvis, as indicated by the title of the book. It is of course better to watch a technique being performed than to read about it, but one has to admit that a book constitutes a ready and convenient piece of reference on which the reader can always dwell. The techniques which have been included are the ones which I have personally found most efficacious after having treated hundreds of patients. It has to be remembered that the application of techniques as described can be modified to suit the manipulator and the patient being manipulated. This is because the details of procedure described reflect my personal approach. Since each individual can evolve his own approach, modification of methods as described is not unexpected so long as the underlying principles are not kept out of focus.

I have tried to get away from a pathology-oriented perspective in my approach toward manipulative treatment of back pain. As a result, I have tried to relate the various methods of examination and technique application to the patient's signs and symptoms rather than to the traditional diagnostic labels. This practical approach steers clear of the polemics which arise when certain diagnostic titles are employed, since there is no consensus yet on this point. We have to wait for the clarification of the pathological uncertainties associated with the common back pain.

An attempt has been made to lead the reader through an interesting path. He will notice that one step leads to another logical and rational step, starting from the Preamble, followed by a review of the History of Manipulation, Anatomy, Examination of the Spine, Technique Application, and so on to the Conclusion.

This book does not present manipulation as a panacea. However, it makes the point that manipulation has a place in the armamentarium of manual therapy. It also has a place among the modalities aimed at reducing human suffering and increasing man's quality of life. The use of heat massage and exercises to relieve back pain is still widely practiced but there are very few people who do not see the inadequacy of this traditional and perhaps anachronistic approach. Spinal manipulation may be able to rectify this inadequacy and make the practitioner more useful to his patient.

Acknowledgments

Many people have contributed to the materialization of a 10-year-old dream which became a reality in the form of this book.

The constructive help and inspiring support of Miss Janis Murphy were particularly welcomed during the writing of this book. Despite her busy schedule as she worked toward her doctorate degree at the University of Minnesota in Minneapolis, she still found time to pose for many of the photographs.

My grateful thanks are due to Miss Kathie Hanson who obligingly acted as model for most of the photographs and for her encouragement and moral support, especially at the early part of the preparation of this book.

I am happy to express my lasting appreciation to Miss Judy Morgan, the Rehabilitation Co-ordinator, Fairview Hospital, Minneapolis, and to her Assistant, Miss Carolyn Woodring for allowing me to take photographs during my brief working period in their department. My thanks to Miss Patty Ness and Miss Lou Ann Nemnich who posed for the photographs taken there.

My special thanks will go to Professor Roy Walmsley, Queen's University, Kingston, Canada, who agreed to read the manuscript and write a Foreword to the book.

I wish to place on record my appreciation of the photographic skill and patience of Mr. Lloyd Weinheimer who took most of the pictures in this book.

I am much indebted to Doctor John Lonstein, orthopedic surgeon, Fairview Hospital, Minneapolis, the True-Eze Manufacturing Company, Burbank, California, and the Editors of *The American Scientist*, New Haven, Connecticut, for supplying me with illustrations and allowing me to use them for the book. My grateful thanks to Geigy Pharmaceutical Company, Basel, Switzerland and to Cassell, Bailliere and Tindall, London, England for allowing me to use illustrations from their publications.

I am unable to express adequately my gratitude to Ms. Sara Finnegan of the Williams & Wilkins Co., Baltimore, Maryland, who patiently and diligently sorted out the many thorny problems which cropped up during the preparation of this book for publication.

To many other people, who by their comments and guidance have contributed to the writing of this book, I hereby express my sincere thanks. They will be thanked in appropriate terms and personally whenever and if they can be found.

Finally, I am humbly conscious of how much this book reflects how much I learned from the many patients who submitted themselves to my hands for manipulation. I owe them the decency of their cooperation as I tried to document factors attendant on back pain and the degree of efficacy of manipulation as a modality in its treatment. To these patients, I give my sincerest gratitude.

V. C. Nwuga
Ile-Ife, Nigeria
1975

Table of Contents

PREFACE vii

ACKNOWLEDGMENTS ix

CHAPTER 1

PREAMBLE 1

CHAPTER 2

A REVIEW OF HISTORY AND SCHOOLS OF THOUGHT 4
Bonesetting
Osteopathy and Chiropractic
Manipulation in Recent Times

CHAPTER 3

ANATOMY AND MECHANICS OF THE SPINAL COLUMN . . . 12
Characteristics of the Vertebrae
Joints
Ligaments
Movements
Surface Anatomy

CHAPTER 4

EXAMINATION OF THE PATIENT 23
Initial Questioning and Observation
History
Pain
Neurological Examination
Gross Spinal Movements
Intervertebral Mobility Tests
Examination of the Sacroiliac Joint
General Consideration and Other Tests

CHAPTER 5

TECHNIQUES OF SPINAL MANIPULATION 47

CHAPTER 6

CLINICAL APPLICATION OF SPINAL MANIPULATION 67
Selection of Techniques
Application of Oscillatory Techniques
Application of Manipulative Thrusts
Vacuum Snaps
Reaction of Patients and Signs and Symptoms to Treatment
Cervical Headaches
Duration and Frequency of Treatment
Recording of Treatments
The Operator/Patient Relationship
Dangers and Contraindications of Manipulation
Prerequisites for a Safe and Successful Manipulation

CHAPTER 7

TRACTION 82
Cervical Traction
Lumbar Traction
Contraindications of Traction

CHAPTER 8

CASE HISTORIES 96

CHAPTER 9

DISCUSSION 109
The Riddle of Back Pain
The Physical Therapist and Manipulation
Educational Opportunities and World Organizations in Manipulative
Therapy
Science versus Chiropractic Philosophy

CHAPTER 10

CONCLUSION 117

chapter 1

Preamble

The problem of pain in the case of the common backache has been such a conundrum that people concerned with its care are still searching for the right solution. The economic cost to the sufferer runs into vast amounts of money but the costs of human discomfort, distress and suffering cannot be calculated in pecuniary terms.

My interest in manipulative therapy started during my undergraduate days as a physiotherapy student at the Royal Herbert Hospital, London, England. I observed with dissatisfaction the treatment of patients who had back and neck pain with the usual traditional modalities at the hospitals with which I was affiliating for practical training. Some of these patients improved but a sizable number either derived a transient relief or none at all. Many of them became despondent and decided to seek relief from their distress by consulting osteopaths and other lay manipulators. I followed up the progress of these patients and discovered to my surprise that their visits to these manipulators paid off. This was a pointer to the gap in my training and I decided to rectify this apparent deficiency.

I started to read every available publication on the subject of manipulation, and after graduation I attended courses and listened to lectures on the subject. This was the beginning of my problems. I soon discovered that this was an area of study laden with legion controversies, confusion of thought, and a large degree of misunderstanding with regard to pathology, rationale behind manipulation, the indications and contraindications and so on.

This book is an attempt to resolve some of the current conflicts, remove the veil of mystique and emotionalism surrounding the subject of manipulation and present the subject in a clearer light.

To many people the word manipulation still conjures up visions of wrenching of joints by osteopaths, forceful maneuvers by chiropractors, forcible movement of joints by orthopedic surgeons with the patient under anesthesia, or at best something resembling a one-sided wrestling match! In many quarters it is even regarded as taboo, a form of treatment which is dangerous and therefore not to be talked about.

These unfortunate and jaundiced views are the results of ignorance and misconceptions of a form of therapy which has proved valuable since time immemorial when properly administered. Manipulation in this context is a skillful form of passive movement administered to a spinal joint with the objectives of relieving pain, and/or spasm, and restoring normal movement and function.

Why has manipulative therapy not been able to enjoy the respect, recognition and pride of place which it deserves? It has to be remembered that the subject is a victim of history. The various negative attitudes which it has faced are relics of the past. Today's attitude is a hangover from the days of bonesetters, Andrew Still who defected from medicine and formulated the osteopathic concept and David Palmer who instituted chiropractic.

The exaggerated claims of the practitioners of this art have exasperated orthodox medicine which has failed to find a scientific basis for those claims. On the other hand, orthodox medicine finds it difficult to admit its own ignorance of the subject for fear of losing face. Very few doctors manipulate and the subject is rarely taught in medical schools. The physiotherapy profession, which traditionally has been guided by medical thought, has always been isolated not only from the practitioners of manipulation but also from the literature pertaining to the subject. A survey which was conducted in the United States in 1970 to find out to what extent manipulative therapy was being taught in physical therapy schools revealed that only 9 out of 51 accredited schools included the subject in one form or another in their curricula.[1] Some of the criticisms of the medical profession may be justified, however, in view of the circumstances and persons who perform this kind of treatment.

The merits and demerits of manipulation should be investigated before any judgments are made. It has to be mentioned, however, that one of the difficulties to be faced in assessing the value of manipulation is that it has both artistic and scientific components. The scientific aspect can be assimilated by anyone interested in the subject, but for some unknown reason, various practitioners seem to vary in their skill of its application.

Much has been said about the dangers of manipulation. This is a reality of course but only when the rules are disregarded and when it is attempted by the uninitiated. But we should not forget too quickly that there are dangers associated with surgery, taking of drugs, dentistry, heat therapy and various other attempts aimed at improving the human condition. It is estimated that 75 million manipulations are performed annually in North America.[2] It will be interesting to compare the number of injuries and resulting litigations from these with those which arise from surgical intervention. Usually it is only the patients who have received injury at the manipulators' hands who are noticed while a blind eye is conveniently turned to the many patients who have been helped. It is only fair that medicine should close this hiatus in its own knowledge before a justified criticism can be leveled at manipulation. The success of chiropractors and osteopaths, even if it is painful and embarrassing to concede, is a testimony that they are doing some kind of good. It is only research which will substantiate this or prove that it is the public who is gullible. Failure to conduct a thorough investigation into the matter will only lead to the continuation of a grateful multitude of irregular practitioners of various stripes and names in the field.

Manipulative therapy is an art based on scientific principles and an intimate knowledge of human anatomy. It entails not brute force, but a logical and persuasive skill. It would be pretentious to say that manipulation is a panacea as it is sometimes claimed. There is nothing wrong with it except probably the present circumstances under which it is performed. Its advocates should descend from their pedestal, adopt a realistic attitude with regard to its virtues so that opponents will no longer have reason to scorn this form of therapy. There is no doubt that it is an effective form of treatment when used by the right person for the appropriate case at the appropriate time. Continued prejudice and its exclusion from the health care scene are a disservice to the patient.

REFERENCES

1. Stephens, B. S. Manipulative therapy in physical therapy curriculum. Phys. Ther., 53: 40–50, 1973.
2. Livingston, M. C. P. Spinal manipulation in medical practice: A century of ignorance. Med. J. Aust., 2: 552–555, 1968.

chapter 2

A review of history and schools of thought

The history of manipulation is lost in the midst of antiquity. It is an art which men and women have practiced on each other since prehistoric times.

The first documentation of manipulation was made by Hippocrates (460 B.C. to 375 B.C.).[1] He taught his students to apply a vertical manipulative thrust on a gibbus (a prominent vertebra) and to give exercises afterward.

4

Galen made reference to the manipulation of the spine for misalignment in a patient following trauma to the neck.[2]

BONESETTING

For many centuries in England, bonesetters practiced manipulation as a family tradition. Bonesetters still exist not only in England but in many European countries. The bonesetter did not set bones in the modern meaning like the surgeon who sets fractures, but people consulted him to have their joints manipulated because they were causing pain.

The bonesetter was invariably an unschooled countryman who learned his profession from his forefather and the trade secrets were confined within the family. The rationale for his treatment was that "a little bone was out of place" and that manipulation could be used to put it back and the patient thus could be relieved of pain.

For a long time orthodox medicine viewed bonesetting as a mysterious art until Dr. Wharton Hood published a treatise entitled, *On Bonesetting*, a pioneer work which received wide acclaim. The way in which this publication became a reality is interesting. It was based on the observations of the work of Richard Hutton, a famous bonesetter of his day who had a practice in the West End of London. Hutton had invited Dr. Peter Hood (Dr. Wharton Hood's father) to watch him and to learn something of his bonesetting techniques. However, it was Dr. Hood, Jr. who accepted the invitation on behalf of his father, who was too busy. This invitation was a reciprocal gesture on the part of Richard Hutton who had been a patient of Peter Hood during a serious illness; after his recovery, the latter had refused to charge him any fees for his services. After the death of Hutton in 1871, Peter Hood published a series of articles in the *Lancet* in England, outlining Hutton's bonesetting techniques.[3] These articles were later published in the form of the treatise, *On Bonesetting*.

In 1867, Sir James Paget (1814 to 1899), the renowned British surgeon, published his famous lecture, "Cases that bonesetters cure" in the *British Medical Journal*.[4] Paget delineated the types of cases which were responsive to manipulative therapy. He exhorted his listeners to "learn them, to imitate what is good and avoid what is bad in the practice of bonesetters." He added that too long a rest was the most frequent cause of delay in recovery in traumatized joints and in the unaffected parts which had been rested because of nearness to the injured part.

However, Paget's injunctions fell on deaf ears. Orthodox medicine of the day found the rationale behind bonesetting untenable, an attitude probably justified in part, even though patients who had visited bonesetters attested to their skill. Armed with an armamentarium of diagnostic tools and having shown scientifically that the "little bone" which the bonesetter mentions does not go out of place, modern medicine is reluctant to go along with such thinking. On the other hand, no scientific explanation has been procured to explain the bonesetter's successes.

OSTEOPATHY AND CHIROPRACTIC

Two major schools of thought which are relatively new in the field of manipulation are osteopathy and chiropractic. Superficially, these two schools bear certain resemblances to each other with regard to the mechanistic approach to illness, but beyond that the philosophies underlying them are different.

The story of chiropractic (Pronounced ki-ro-prak'-tik) began in Davenport, Iowa with Daniel David Palmer. Palmer was born in Port Perry, Ontario in 1845. In 1895 he reported that he "cured" the deafness of a black janitor, Henry Lillard, after he "adjusted" the latter's misaligned vertebra. Palmer's belief was that the spinal column was the controller of the human machinery, and that all diseases could be traced to it.

Palmer founded the first chiropractic school in Davenport in 1897. Since then, it has been reported that over 500 chiropractic institutions have operated at one time or another in the United States.[5] Today there are 14 chiropractic colleges in the United States recognized by the two major chiropractic professional associations—the National Chiropractic Association (N.C.A.), founded in 1910, and the International Chiropractic Association (I.C.A.), founded in 1926.

The chiropractic profession in the United States supports two major diagnostic and therapeutic philosophical schools. One school is a firm adherent to the original teachings of Palmer and leans heavily on the use of manual adjustments of the spine in its therapeutic approach. The followers of this tradition are called "straights." The other school of thought utilizes electrical treatments, dietary regime and other modalities as adjuncts to manual adjustments. These practitioners are called "mixers."

The basis of chiropractic philosophy is the theory of "subluxation." Chiropractors claim that subluxation in the spinal column interferes with nerve function and that this is the significant factor in disease causation. Manipulation of the appropriate area of the spine restores the natural alignment of the spine which in turn relieves the symptoms. Statements regarding the adjustment of the spine for conditions such as diabetes, various intestinal disorders, heart trouble and cancer are quite common in chiropractic literature.

The history of osteopathy is intimately connected with Andrew Taylor Still (1828 to 1917).[6] He was osteopathy's progenitor. Still was the son of a pioneer Methodist doctor and he studied medicine at the College of Physicians and Surgeons in Kansas City, Missouri.

Following the end of the Civil War in which he fought as a major, Still lost three of his sons in an epidemic of spinal meningitis, even though they had had the best medical treatment available. Still became disillusioned with orthodox medicine as it was practiced during his day. A deeply religious man, the idea of osteopathy came to Still like a revelation. He concluded that the human body possessed self-healing properties, that efficient functioning was dependent on unimpaired structure and that proper nerve and blood supply to the tissues was necessary for health maintenance. These concepts were contained in his *Rule of the Artery* which he enunciated in 1874 and which became the basic concept of osteopathy. He exhumed the bodies of dead Indians and studied the skeletal system until he became an expert in this area. His intimate knowledge of the skeletal system and the tragic loss of his sons probably were powerful factors directing his thought processes in the formulation of the osteopathic philosophy for disease causation.

One must view Andrew Still in the background of medicine as it was then practiced in the Midwestern part of the United States. It was far from satisfactory. His alienation therefore has to be interpreted against this perspective. He was dissatisfied with a system of therapy which consisted of "pouring drugs about which he knew little into bodies about which he knew less." [7]

He observed that certain headaches often occurred concurrently with tenderness in the cervical region. He noted movement limitations in certain areas, manipulation of which relieved the symptoms. His diagnosis of these tender spots in the spine was "osteopathic lesion." These spots, however, were regarded by his allopathic colleagues as visceral disease. This probably was a situation in which brachial neuralgia caused by a cervical spondylosis was confused with pain of angina extending down the arm.[8] With admirable ingenuity, Still worked out a system of manipulations designed to rectify functional bony deviations in the body.

The medical profession was not impressed. Still was determined to disseminate this new-found knowledge, however, and founded the American School of Osteopathy in 1892 in Kirksville, Missouri.

Today, osteopaths consider their discipline a considerable refinement and modification of Still's original ideas. In their approach, the modern osteopaths view the human frame with a holistic perspective, using what modality they think is appropriate, although there is some emphasis on the mechanistic approach. They employ all scientifically based medical and surgical techniques in addition to manipulations. Because it has discarded some of its pristine shibboleths and conceded the fallibility of some of its Stillerian tenets, osteopathy has been accepted as a bona fide system of healing by orthodox medicine in many but not all quarters. In many instances, organized medicine has bent over backward to make concessions to osteopathy. In 1962 over 2000 licensed osteopaths in the state of California received the Doctor of Medicine degree with the approbation of the California Medical Association, and the State Osteopathic College became converted into a fully accredited medical school.[9]

Today in the United States, 41 states including the District of Columbia extend the same type of legal rights to doctors of osteopathy (D.O.s) to care for all diseases and ailments as doctors of medicine (M.D.s). Osteopathy now seems to be merging back into medicine from which it defected about 100 years ago.

By sharp contrast, the chiropractor is still regarded as an outcast, although a successful one.[10] His inability to explain his rationale for treatment in accepted scientific terms or to justify his concepts has run him into problems with orthodox medicine. This situation will remain the same as long as chiropractic attitudes are frozen in the Palmerian inspiration.

Since the back is the focus of attention, the chiropractor often makes a thorough clinical and radiological examination of this area. This includes full length X-ray pictures of the spine—antero-posterior and lateral views. This liberal use of X-rays has generated concern in the scientific community in view of the radiation to which chiropractic patients are exposed. However, the X-ray examination is one of the chiropractor's selling points.[11] Even though it inflates the cost of chiropractic care, it protects the chiropractor medico-legally; it is also convincing and impressive to the patient.

MANIPULATION IN RECENT TIMES

At the moment there is still no consensus as to the rationale behind spinal manipulations, but there exists a wealth of theories. Each school of thought has advanced its own rationale and evolved manipulative techniques consistent with it. Much controversy still surrounds the question of the origin of pain in the common backache. Does the pain emanate from the intervertebral disc, the dura or apophyseal joint? How does spinal manipulation bring about relief? These are questions with long overdue answers.

James Mennell, who was once in charge of the Physical Medicine Department at St. Thomas' Hospital in London, published a book in 1952 entitled *The Science and Art of Joint Manipulation*.[12] He pointed to the facet joints, postural strain and adhesions as causative factors in back pain. Later, his son John enunciated the concepts of "joint play" and "joint dysfunction." [13, 14] Joint play refers to the involuntary movement which occurs concurrently with the gross voluntary movement. The integrity of the voluntary movement hinges on the integrity of the voluntary joint play movement. Loss of joint play as occurs in traumatic cases and diseases precipitates a situation of joint dysfunction. As an extension of Mennell's theory, the loss of height of the intervertebral discs with the consequent "misalignment" of the facet joints in advancing age might be a significant pain-producing factor in middle-aged subjects who throng physical therapy departments daily with neck and back pain. Mennell's manipulations are designed to restore joint play for the relief of pain, and for restoration of normal voluntary movement and function.

In 1933, Mixter and Barr presented a paper to the annual meeting of the New England Surgical Society in Boston. It was published as an article in the *New England Journal of Medicine* in 1934.[15] Today it is regarded as a classic. In it Mixter and Barr pointed an accusing finger at the intervertebral disc as a major factor in backache with or without sciatica. Their momentous work has had a powerful effect on medical thought since then, stimulating much interest and leading to a series of excellent publications on the subject.[16-21]

Prominent among those who subscribe to the disc school of thought is James Cyriax who, before his retirement, was the orthopedic physician at St. Thomas' Hospital in London, after James Mennell. More than any physician, he has done a great deal to bring the usefulness of manipulation to the attention of the medical profession. His book, *Textbook of Orthopaedic Medicine*, first published in 1954, is invaluable.[22] Because of his ardent belief in the disc as a source of back pain problems, most of Cyriax' manipulative techniques are designed for the reduction of disc herniation.[23] Cyriax identifies two types of disc lesion. The first is due to nuclear protrusion characterized by gradual onset with gradual increase in pain, occurring more among younger patients. The second type is due to annular protrusion and is more amenable to manipulative reduction.

Cyriax claims that his rotatory maneuvers apply a torsional stress on the spine. This exerts a centripetal force which reduces the prolapsed or bulging disc material if the longitudinal ligaments are intact.[24]

Much criticism has been leveled at Cyriax because of the massive tractive force he applies while manipulating and because of the non-specificity of many of his techniques. However, most authorities agree that his techniques of examination prior to manipulation are superb and contain a wealth of medical logic. It is especially for this that he will be remembered.

A school of thought which has attracted some attention especially in Europe is being led by Robert Maigne, who has postulated the "concept of painlessness and opposite motion." [25-27] This concept states that a manipulative maneuver should be administered in the direction opposite to the movement that is restricted and causing pain. For example, limitation of spinal movement to the left can be rectified by a maneuver which involves rotation to the right. Maigne distinguishes between "mobilizations" and "manipulations." The former refers to a series of passive movements administered within the available range of movement without going beyond it. The latter involves a sudden low amplitude thrust which goes beyond the limited range of movement. This maneuver takes the joint beyond its voluntary and usual range but the joint stays within its anatomic limit. Maigne, like Cyriax, has worked hard to focus medical attention on manipulative therapy as an effective modality in the relief of pain.

In France is a less well known group of medical practitioners who combine osteopathic and chiropractic philosophies in their approach toward manipulation. Their rationale for manipulation is that a lesion in the spine changes the efferent nerve impulses with undesirable effects on the organs to which these impulses are destined. This sets up a vicious cycle causing atrophy and malfunction in the affected part, and then in the spine, and so on. Manipulative therapy is often used to adjust the spine as an adjunct to other therapeutic procedures.

The driving force behind a school of thought which has flourished in Scandinavia is Kaltenborn, who is a physiotherapist, as well as chiropractor and an osteopath. Due to his immense efforts, charismatic personality and high quality expertise, he has earned the respect of doctors in Norway who have helped his attempts to seek expansion of the charter of physiotherapists in Norway to include manipulative therapy. This materialized in 1957 with the approval of the Norwegian Health Authorities, and led to the inauguration of an association of physiotherapists specializing in manipulation in the same year. An organization of doctors interested in the subject was formed in 1962. In an attempt to spread the word, Kaltenborn has taught courses to doctors and physiotherapists in Sweden, Denmark, Iceland and in his native Norway. Participants come from all over the world, especially from Europe. His work has led to a revolution in thinking among medical men in Scandinavia and in many parts of the world.

The philosophy behind Kaltenborn's techniques is a fusion of what he has considered the best in chiropractic, osteopathy and physical medicine. He uses Cyriax' methods (which he learned at St. Thomas' Hospital, London, in 1952) to evaluate the patient and employs mainly specific osteopathic and sometimes chiropractic techniques for treatment. He sees strain as the basis of pathology in joints. The resulting inflammation and edema cause pressure on nerves resulting in pain and spasm.[28] The spasm increases pain and a vicious cycle is set up. Edematous thickenings arise later causing joint restriction and lack of mobility. This process can occur either in the spinal or peripheral joints. He therefore finds it expedient to manipulate the joint when there is evidence of altered mobility before the cycle is initiated, or if it has, to break it.

In 1964 Maitland published his book, *Vertebral Manipulation*.[29] Like Maigne[25-27] he distinguishes between mobilization and manipulation but puts heavy emphasis on mobilization. His techniques are fairly similar to the "articulatory" techniques used by osteopaths, involving oscillatory movements performed on a chosen joint in which the movement induced by the therapist is within the patient's available range of movement tolerance in order to release a fixed synovial joint. Maitland does not seem interested in the flurry of controversy surrounding the rationale behind manipulative techniques. He is merely interested in physical signs for which he applies the appropriate manipulative techniques. Because his techniques are of a gentle nature and easier to learn, they have appealed to physiotherapists and have gained much recognition especially in Australia (where Maitland is a private practitioner in physiotherapy and a part-time tutor at the University of Adelaide) and in the United Kingdom. By using the word mobilization instead of manipulation, he has successfully eliminated the emotional heat surrounding the subject, which has led to better acceptance of the subject among members of the medical profession.

REFERENCES

1. *Massage, Manipulation and Traction*, (Licht, S., Ed.) Physical Medicine Library, vol. V. New Haven, Connecticut, 1960.
2. Drummer, T. G. and Mahe, A. *Out on the Fringe* (translated from French). Parrish, London, 1963.
3. Fisher, A. G. T. *Treatment by Manipulation*. H. K. Lewis and Co., London, 1948.
4. Paget, Sir James. Cases that bonesetters cure. Br. Med. J., *1:* 1–4, 1867.
5. McClusky, T. *Your Health and Chiropractic*. Milestone Books, New York, 1964.
6. Booth, E. R. *History of Osteopathy*. Canton Press, Cincinnati, Ohio, 1924.
7. Still, A. T. *Autobiography*. Kirksville, Missouri, 1908.
8. Symposium. Manipulative treatment. Med. J. Aust., *1:* 1274–1280, 1967.
9. Inglis, B. *Fringe Medicine*. Faber and Faber, London, 1964.
10. Rowland, G. A. The successful outcast. Pa. Med., *75:* 20, 1972.
11. Ebbetts, J. The chiropractic physician looks at the lumbar intervertebral disc. Paper read at the British Association of Manipulative Medicine Symposium on Diagnosis and Treatment of Intervertebral Disc Prolapse, March, 1970.
12. Mennell, J. *The Science and Art of Joint Manipulation,* vol. II. J. and A. Churchill, London, 1952.
13. Mennell, J. *Back Pain*. Little Brown, Boston, 1960.
14. Mennell, J. *Joint Pain*. Little Brown, Boston, 1964.
15. Mixter, W. J. and Barr, J. S. Rupture of the intervertebral disc with involvement of the spinal canal. New Engl. J. Med., *211:* 210–215, 1934.
16. Dandy, W. E. Concealed ruptured intervertebral discs: Plea for elimination of contrast medium in diagnosis. J. A. M. A., *117:* 820–823, 1941.
17. Key, J. A. Intervertebral disc lesions are the most common cause of low back pain with or without sciatica. Ann. Surg., *121:* 534–544, 1945.
18. Burns, B. H. and Young, R. H. Protrusion of intervertebral disc. Lancet, *2:* 424–427, 1945.
19. Lindblom, K. Experimental ruptures of intervertebral discs in rats tails. J. Bone Joint Surg., *34A:* 123–128, 1952.
20. Jonck, L. M. The mechanical disturbances from lumbar disc space narrowing. J. Bone Joint Surg., *43B:* 362–375, 1961.
21. Armstrong, J. R. Lumbar Disc Lesions. E. and S. Livingstone, London, 1965.
22. Cyriax, J. *Textbook of Orthopaedic Medicine,* vol. I. Williams & Wilkins, Baltimore, 1969.
23. Cyriax, J. *Textbook of Orthopaedic Medicine,* vol. II. Williams & Wilkins, Baltimore, 1965.
24. Cyriax, J. Correspondence. Br. Med. J., *4:* 133, 1969.
25. Maigne, R. *Les Manipulations Vertebrales*. Expansion Scientifique, Française, Paris, 1960.
26. Maigne, R. The concept of painlessness and opposite motion in spinal manipulations (translated from French). Am. J. Phys. Med., *44:* 55–69, 1965.
27. Maigne, R. Le choix des manipulations dans le traitement des sciatiques. Rev. Rheum., *32:* 366–372, 1965.
28. Brodin, H., Bang, J., Bechgarrd, P., Kaltenborn, F. and Schoitz, E. *Manipulation av Ryggraden*. Scandinavicen University Books, 1966.
29. Maitland, G. D. *Vertebral Manipulation*. Butterworth, London, 1964.

chapter 3

Anatomy and mechanics of the spinal column

Before the numerous subtleties and the various problems attendant on spinal manipulation can be understood, it is mandatory that the manipulative therapist understand the components which constitute the spine, including the mechanical interaction taking place between these components. It cannot be overemphasized that one needs to have an accurate mental picture of the particular joint which one is trying to influence at any one time during manipulation. When this is lacking, the therapist will only be groping in the dark and his treatment will be ineffectual.

The purpose of this chapter is to lay out the basic points of the anatomy and mechanics of the spine. It is intended to refresh the memory of the reader. It is by no means comprehensive. More detailed information, if desired, can be obtained from available anatomy textbooks.

The spinal column constitutes the core of the locomotor apparatus and is the key to the posture of the trunk. It transmits the weight of the upper portions of the body, provides a stable central point for the attachment of bones and muscles of the upper and lower limbs and serves as an excellent shield for the spinal cord with its adjacent spinal nerves.

The spinal column is made up of 33 vertebrae which are labeled according to the regions of the body in which they are found. There are thus seven cervical, 12 thoracic, five sacral and four coccygeal vertebrae. Lying between the vertebrae are pads of fibrocartilage, the intervertebral discs. The spinal cord passes through a vertebral canal, the vertebral foramen formed by the vertebrae. This foramen is triangular and large in the cervical and lumbar regions while assuming a somewhat small and circular shape in the thoracic region. The intervertebral foramina, which are openings between adjacent vertebrae, give passage to the paired spinal nerves which convey impulses to and from the spinal cord. These foramina are smallest in the cervical region and become larger in size toward the lower lumbar vetebrae.

When the spine is viewed from the side (Figure 3.1) the cervical and lumbar regions exhibit a forward convexity, while the thoracic and pelvic curves are concave forward. The cervical curve starts with the first cervical vertebra and ends at the fifth cervical vertebra. The most prominent point on the thoracic curve is at the level of the seventh thoracic vertebra. The lumbar curve ends at the lumbo-sacral angle while the pelvic curve commences at the lumbo-sacral angle and ends at the tip of the coccyx.

CHARACTERISTICS OF THE VERTEBRAE

The vertebrae are basically similar with the exception of the atlas and axis.

A typical vertebra (Figure 3.2) consists essentially of two parts, the anteriorly placed body and the neural arch. Together these make up the walls of the vertebral foramen. The body of the vertebra which is its thickest part gives attachment to the intervertebral discs on its flat superior and inferior surfaces. Piercing the body are a few small foramina which provide passage for nutrient vessels.

The neural arch is made up of two pedicles and two laminae which give rise to seven processes. The pedicles are short and thick and originate from the postero-lateral aspects of the body. The laminae are broad and flat and extend posteriorly and medially from the ends of the pedicles. The spinous process projects posteriorly from the meeting point of the two laminae. At the point where the laminae and pedicles meet, the trans-

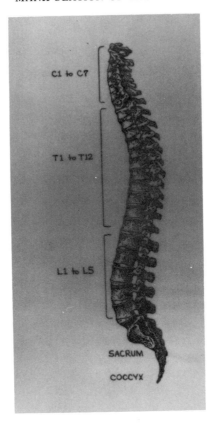

FIG. 3.1. Left side view of the spinal column.

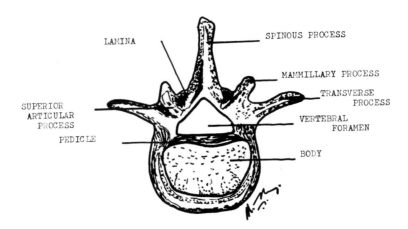

FIG. 3.2. Diagrammatic view of a typical lumbar vertebra.

verse process projects laterally. There are four articular processes, two superior and two inferior, and they originate from the meeting point of the pedicles and the laminae. A layer of hyaline cartilage covers the surfaces of the articular processes.

The vertebrae vary in their shape and size in the different regions of the vertebral column. The lumbar vertebrae which support the weight of the trunk are larger than the cervical vertebrae which comparatively have to contend with the weight of the skull. The vertebral bodies and transverse processes in the thoracic region are provided with additional facets for the costo-vertebral articulations.

The first cervical vertebra, the atlas, resembles a ring-like bony structure and it provides a resting seat for the skull (Figure 3.3). Its striking feature is that it has no vertebral body and it consists of two lateral masses which are joined anteriorly and posteriorly by arches. The superior surfaces

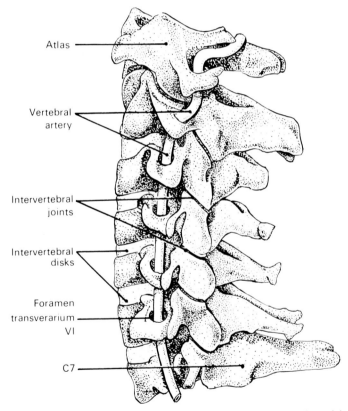

Atlas

Vertebral artery

Intervertebral joints

Intervertebral disks

Foramen transverarium VI

C7

FIG. 3.3. Cervical vertebrae in the adult viewed from the side. Reproduced from Krayenbühl, H. and Zander, E. Rupture of lumbar and cervical intervertebral disks. Documenta Rheumatologica Geigy No. 1, 1956, Basel. By permission of the publishers CIBA-GEIGY Limited, Basel, Switzerland.

of the lateral masses are provided with facets which articulate with the occipital condyles of the skull. The facets on the inferior surface of the lateral masses articulate with the second cervical vertebra, the axis. The transverse processes are pierced by oval-shaped foramina which provide passage for the vertebral artery and its accompanying vein and nerve.

The second cervical vertebra, the axis, can be readily recognized by its prominent odontoid process which projects vertically upward from its body. The spinous process on its posterior aspect is large and bifid. Its superior articular facet makes it possible for the axis to form an articulation with the axis, while it articulates with the third cervical vertebra below through its inferior articular facet. Like the atlas, the transverse

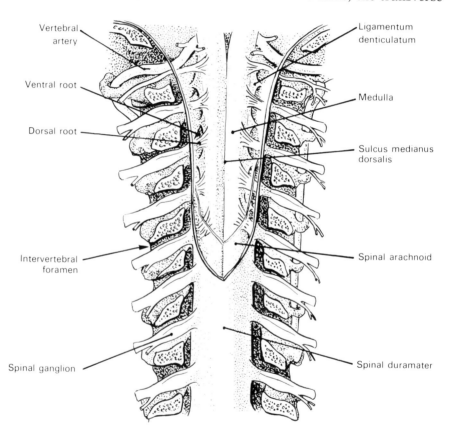

Vertebral artery · Ventral root · Dorsal root · Intervertebral foramen · Spinal ganglion · Ligamentum denticulatum · Medulla · Sulcus medianus dorsalis · Spinal arachnoid · Spinal duramater

FIG. 3.4. Topography of the spinal cord and cervical nerves. The vertebral arches have been removed and the upper part of the dura mater opened.

Reproduced from Krayenbühl, H. and Zander, E. Rupture of lumbar and cervical intervertebral disks. Documenta Rheumatologica Geigy No. 1, 1956, Basel. By permission of the publishers CIBA-GEIGY Limited, Basel, Switzerland.

processes are equipped with foramina for the passage of the vertebral artery and its accompanying vein and nerve.

JOINTS

The main joints of the vertebral column are the symphyses between the bodies of adjacent vertebrae and the joints between the inferior and superior articular processes.

Atlanto-Occipital Joints

These result from the articulation between the facets on the lateral mass of the first cervical vertebra and the occipital condyles placed at the base of the skull.

Atlanto-Axial Joints

There are three points of articulation between the first and second cervical vertebrae. One of these is the articulation between the posterior part of the anterior arch of the first cervical vertebra and the anterior part of the odontoid process of the second vertebra; the others are the two paired facet articulations between the two vertebrae in question.

Facet-Joints

These are sometimes referred to as either the "posterior joints," the "zygapophyseal joints" or the "apophyseal joints." They are the result of the articulation between the superior and inferior articular processes originating from the vertebral arches of adjacent vertebrae. These joints are diathrodial in nature and are complete with synovial membrane and joint capsule. The capsule displays a laxity which allows a free range of gliding movement to take place. The facet joints in the cervical region are arranged in a coronal plane; so also are those in the lumbo-sacral joint. Those in the thoracic and lumbar regions are approximately in the sagittal plane. The function of the facet joints is to stabilize the spine. The planes of the articular surfaces are designed in such a way as to allow movement while simultaneously disallowing forward displacement of the vertebrae on each other. In this way they control movement between adjacent vertebrae and place a restriction on the movements which do not take place along their planes.

Costovertebral Joints

These joints are made by 12 pairs of ribs which form an articulation with the thoracic spinal column through the heads of the ribs with the bodies of the thoracic vertebrae and the transverse processes. The two facets on the head of the rib form an articulation with the lateral aspect of the adjacent vertebral bodies. In addition, a third facet on the neck of the rib articulates with the transverse process of the vertebra which corresponds to it numerically.

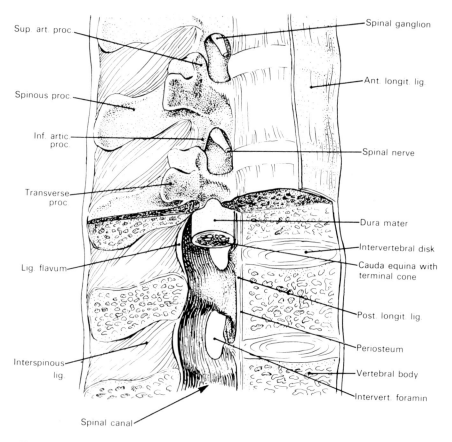

Sup. art. proc.

Spinous proc.

Inf. artic. proc

Transverse proc

Lig. flavum

Interspinous lig.

Spinal canal

Spinal ganglion

Ant. longit. lig

Spinal nerve

Dura mater

Intervertebral disk

Cauda equina with terminal cone

Post. longit. lig

Periosteum

Vertebral body

Intervert. foramin

FIG. 3.5 Diagrammatic view of the lumbar spine and the spinal cord. Reproduced from Krayenbühl, H. and Zander, E. Rupture of lumbar and cervical intervertebral disks. Documenta Rheumatologica Geigy No. 1, 1956, Basel. By permission of the publishers CIBA-GEIGY Limited, Basel, Switzerland.

Sacroiliac Joint

This is an articulation between the auricular surface of the sacrum and the corresponding articular surface on the ilium. The sacroiliac joint displays a dual structure, part fibrous and part synovial.

LIGAMENTS

Running the length of the spinal column are the anterior and posterior longitudinal ligaments which are distributed in front and back, respectively. The ligamentum flavum lies between adjacent laminae. Because of its elastic nature, it helps to bring the spine back into the position of extension from flexion. The ligamentum flavum also acts in a protective capacity for the spinal cord by the completion of the spinal canal posteriorly. The interspinous ligaments connect adjacent spinous processes while the supraspinous ligaments run over the tips of the spinous processes, connecting them this way. The supraspinous ligament enlarges in the cervical region to become the thick ligamentum nuchae.

In the sacroiliac joints there are the anterior and posterior sacroiliac ligaments. Their positions are indicated by their names. There are also the sacrotuberous ligament, sacrospinous ligament and the iliolumbar ligament.

The intervertebral discs are positioned between the bodies of the presacral segments of the spinal column. The spaces which the discs occupy add up to $1/4$ to $1/5$ of the total length of the spine. The spinal secondary curves (cervical and lumbar) are largely a result of the shape of the discs. The intervertebral disc is essentially made up of the annulus fibrosus and the nucleus pulposus. The annulus comprises successive concentric lamellae of fibers of fibrocartilage. It plays a role in the stability of the spine by binding the vertebral bodies together. It also functions as a retaining envelope for the nucleus. The nucleus which is turgid in nature functions as a fulcrum for vertebral movements and equalizes stresses which fall on the spine. Together the annulus and the nucleus work as shock absorbers, disseminate force in the spine and in the process dampen the insults to which the spine is constantly subjected in functional activities. The cartilaginous end-plates shield the vertebral bodies from the stress which results from weight transmission. They also act as a medium through which fluid is diffused between the intervertebral discs and the vertebral bodies.

MOVEMENTS

An appreciation of the types of movement which occur in the various parts of the spinal column will lead to a better understanding of what movements to look for during examination of the spine which will be discussed in the next chapter. It will also help the manipulative therapist to comprehend the limitations and possibilities of movement in a particular joint under manipulation.

In the occipito-atlantal joint, the principal movements are flexion and extension, whereas in the atlanto-axial joint, it is rotation, although some flexion and extension are detectable.

Neither rotation nor side-flexion in its pure sense is detectable anywhere in the spine, with the exception of the thoraco-lumbar region and it is only possible if the spine is in slight flexion. The reason for this is that as the spine goes into side-flexion the facets of the vertebrae come into apposition thus forcing the vertebrae toward a rotatory direction.

Rotatory movement of the vertebral bodies will occur in the same direction as side-flexion. This rule obtains in the thoracic and lumbar regions only if the movement is initiated from an original position of flexion. However if the original position was from the extended or neutral position, then rotary movement of the vertebral bodies will occur in the opposite direction to which the trunk is side-flexed.

When the spinal column moves in a rotatory direction, a large part of the rotation takes place in the atlanto-axial joint and thoracic regions (Figure 3.6). Actually, during rotation of the cervical spine a large part of this movement takes place in the lower cervical segments and in the lumbar region (with the exception of the area between the lumbar region and the sacrum) rotation is highly limited.

When the spine moves toward the side-flexed position, practically all of the movement takes place in the cervical and lumbar regions (Figure 3.7). This movement is highly restricted in the thoracic region because of the articulations of the ribs to the vertebral elements and the sternum.

Some flexion and extension take place in the thoracic spine but most occur in the cervical and lumbar regions, especially in the latter. These movements take place about a transverse axis which passes through the discs.

The types of movement which occur in the sacroiliac joint have been subjected to much controversy. In women, maximal movement occurs during pregnancy because of increased elasticity of the ligaments of the joint. At the best of times, one requires highly sensitive fingers to detect the minute movements which take place in this joint. Young delineates

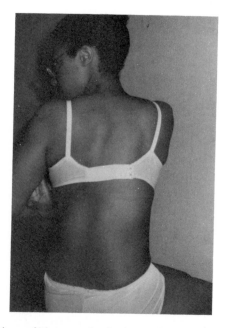

FIG. 3.6. Rotation of the cervical, thoracic and lumbar regions of the spine. Most of the movement takes place in the thoracic region, at the atlanto-occipital and atlanto-axial joints.

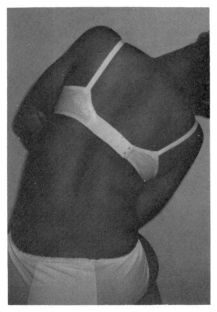

FIG. 3.7. Side flexion of the cervical, thoracic and lumbar regions of the spine. Most of the movement takes place in the cervical and lumbar spines. Note the movement restriction in the thoracic region.

two such kinds of movements.[1] They are of a rotatory and hinge-like nature. His study indicates a downward and upward movement of 2 millimeters in the symphysis pubis in each direction among pregnant women during alternate weight-bearing on one leg at a time. The studies of Brooke,[2] Pittkin[3] and Weist[4] show dissimilar results regarding the point where movement actually occurs. Bourdillon has suggested that the most significant movement of the sacroiliac joint is the antagonistic movement of the ilia about the symphysis pubis.[5] This movement occurs normally during ambulation in a subject with mobile sacroiliac joints.

SURFACE ANATOMY

The easiest structures to palpate in the spine are the spinous processes. When a particular segmental level is identified, the location of other levels can be effected by counting in a proximal or distal direction to the desired level. The seventh cervical vertebra (vertebra prominens), the 11th thoracic vertebra and the fifth lumbar vertebra can best be utilized for this purpose.

The transverse process of the atlas can be located by palpation between the ramus of the mandible and the mastoid process.

The spinous process of the axis can be palpated just below the occiput. Since it is large and is the first palpable suboccipital bony structure it is easy to locate. The transverse process lies below the transverse process of the atlas deep to the sternocleidomastoid muscle.

When running the palpating fingers from the proximal to the distal direction on the neck region, the spinous process of the seventh cervical vertebra is the first that can be easily palpated after that of the second cervical vertebra. It is sometimes difficult to decide whether one is palpating the sixth or seventh cervical vertebra. A differentiation test can easily be performed by placing the head and neck into the extended position while simultaneously placing the palpating fingers on the spinous processes of the sixth and seventh vertebrae. During neck extension, the tip of one of the vertebrae will be found to move forward making palpation difficult. It is invariably the sixth cervical vertebra which behaves in this fashion.

The inferior margin of the articular process of a vertebra can be located just lateral to the corresponding spinous process of the same vertebra and the facet joint. The location of the vertebral transverse process requires a deep palpation since it is buried deep in the muscle.

The spinous process of the third thoracic vertebra is located on the same level as the spine of the scapula. The apex of the scapula is at the level of the spinous process of the vertebra prominens. These guides hold true only if the arms are hanging down at the sides.

It has to be noted that the thoracic spinous processes do not all point at a constant angle. Starting from proximal to distal, they incline downward and this tendency toward inclination increases as far as the seventh or eighth thoracic vertebra. Because of this, the spinous processes and transverse processes do not correspond to each other numerically. Thus for example, the fourth thoracic vertebra is in the same horizontal level as the transverse process of the fifth thoracic vertebra, and the spinous process of the eighth thoracic vertebra lies in the same level as the ninth or 10th thoracic transverse process.

In the lumbar region, the iliac crest lies in the same horizontal level as the spinous process of the fourth lumbar vertebra. This rule does not apply in some subjects whose iliac crests are on the same level as the fith lumbar vertebra.

Using the body of the second sacral vertebra as a guide, it is possible to locate the posterior iliac spines, since they are all usually on the same horizontal level.

REFERENCES

1. Young, J. Relaxation of the pelvic joints in pregnancy. J. Obstet. Gynaecol. Br. Emp., *47:* 493, 1940.
2. Brooke, R. The sacroiliac joint. J. Anat., *58:* 299–305, 1924.
3. Pittkin, H. C. and Pheasant, H. C. Sacrathrogenic telalgia. J. Bone Joint Surg., *18:* 111–133, 365–374, 1936.
4. Weist, H. Movement of the sacroiliac joint. Acta Anat., *23:* 80–91, 1955.
5. Bourdillon, J. F. *Spinal Manipulation.* William Heinemann Medical Books Ltd., London, 1970.

chapter 4
Examination of the patient

Examination of the patient is of paramount importance prior to the administration of manipulative therapy. The ability to observe the patient unobtrusively, to listen attentively to the history and to interpret the signs and symptoms which the patient presents constitutes a prerequisite for a successful treatment. It is this pre-treatment examination of the patient which helps the examiner to formulate a basis and an intelligent rationale for his therapeutic plan. From the author's experience, a first-time examination of the patient usually lasts an average of 20 to 30 minutes compared with the post-examination treatment which lasts an average of 10 minutes. This favorably disproportionate time spent on examination will probably illustrate its importance.

The questions arise. Why does the examiner have to spend so much time examining the patient? Is this really necessary? What exactly are the things he is looking for? What is he going to do with the information which he gleans from this exercise? The answers to these questions are contained in the reasons for examination which are outlined below.

1. Examination of the patient will help the operator to make a choice of the appropriate technique to utilize in treating him. It will also help the operator to avoid the kinds of techniques which will either exacerbate or alter the patient's symptoms one way or the other. During the questioning, if the patient indicates that prone-lying or side-lying on the right increases his pain, it is improbable that his symptoms will be improved by those positions.

2. Examination will lead to a fairly accurate prognostication as to how the patient will react to manipulative treatment. For instance, a patient who has had back pain for many years will take longer to help compared with another whose pain is of recent onset. A patient whose straight-leg-raising is 50 degrees is more likely to have a better prognosis than one whose straight-leg-raising is only 10 degrees. And a patient whose onset of symptoms was sudden and was associated with a particular spinal movement will probably respond better to treatment than one with an insidious and spontaneous onset. These kinds of information will therefore help the examiner to plan treatment accordingly in terms of frequency of treatment and the formulation of treatment goals.

3. The clinical findings during examination will help to determine if manipulation is indicated or contraindicated. When the patient presents certain signs which may indicate some serious illness or certain movement patterns which raise the examiner's suspicion, he should discuss the case with the referring physician and a consensus should be reached with regard to the line of treatment. It is true that before the patient arrives at the therapist's door he would have already been screened by the referring physician. On the other hand, a patient who is not suitable for manipulative treatment sometimes escapes the physician's net. Differential diagnosis in the case of back pain is such a complex matter and the problem of human error is a reality. The author remembers a patient who was referred for "evaluation and manipulation." The diagnosis was "acute lumbar disc syndrome." On examination the articular signs were not consistent with the kinds of picture often encountered. The movements of the spine did not affect the patient's back pain in any way. This patient's condition was later rediagnosed as carcinoma of the bronchus with pain reference to the back. This type of incident does not happen often but one should be aware of its possible occurrence.

4. A thorough clinical assessment will establish a pre-treatment picture of the patient. A comparison with the post-treatment picture will give the examiner a definite idea as to whether the patient has improved or whether his condition has remained static or even deteriorated. For instance, if before treatment the patient had a shooting pain down the gluteal region when he coughed and this disappeared after treatment, it is a positive indication that the patient's condition is showing signs of

improvement. Pre-treatment examination can be likened to the perform-ance of a volitional muscle test, for instance, on the quadriceps after removal of the leg from a plaster cast. The test result constitutes a baseline from which the effects of exercise therapy can be later assessed.

5. A methodical examination will lead the therapist to the exact loca-tion of the patient's lesion. By getting to the source of the pain, the patient is more likely to be helped maximally, thus avoiding waste of the patient's and therapist's time.

It is assumed at this point that the importance of examination has been given enough emphasis. The rest of this chapter will attempt to delineate just what the examiner will be looking for in the examination room and in some cases the significance of certain observations will be outlined.

INITIAL QUESTIONING AND OBSERVATION

Examination of the patient commences when the patient enters the examination room. The overall picture which he presents should be noted. Does he have a good posture? A limp? As he tries to sit down, does he do it easily or is this simple exercise labored and accompanied by wincing and other tell-tale signs of pain? The attitude which he brings into the treatment situation and the non-verbal cues which he gives should be noted and the appropriate communication style adopted.

The patient's age, occupation, hobbies and sports interests should be noted. Younger people respond differently compared with older subjects when treated with manipulative therapy. The kind of work the patient does or his sports activities might give an indication as to the mechanics of an injury to the back. A laborer who spends all day shoveling and lifting, a farmer who is working with heavy equipment or a mother who has a habit of lifting her baby incorrectly might give vital clues as to how their respective pains came about.

When the patient exposes his back, it is observed for excessive lordosis, thoracic kyphosis, scoliosis and general spinal posture. These will give the examiner an insight into the mechanical efficiency of the spine and the kinds of stresses with which the back has to cope. An exaggerated thoracic kyphosis for instance will lead to the contracture of anterior spinal structures, or stretching of the posterior structures and a disturb-ance of costo-vertebral mechanics. In the case of lumbar lordosis, there is excessive compression of the spinal apophyseal joints. There is increased compression of the side of the concavity of the curve presented by a scoliotic spine. In addition, there is osteophyte formation in old cases, ligamentous stretching on the convex side, narrowing of joint spaces and sclerosis of bone on the concave side.

When examining the general spinal posture for any possible devia-tions, the furrow which runs down the center of the back may not give the examiner an accurate picture. For instance some scoliotic conditions have a greater rotatory component than lateral component and a cursory view of the spinous process may not reveal the exact degree of the spinal deformity. If the patient is asked to flex the spine forward the symmetry of the two sides of the back can be assessed by a horizontal view or a tangential view from above. If a scoliosis is present, one side of the back will demonstrate greater upward prominence than the other (Figure 4.1B). When the scoliotic condition is structural in nature, it presents the higher side on the convexity of the curve. If a rotatory component is present in the deformity, a rib hump makes its presence felt as the patient flexes forward.

With the examiner looking at the patient's back, the posterior superior iliac spines can be checked for horizontal alignment. In the standing position the posterior superior iliac spines are indicated by the two dimples in the lower back. During forward flexion the dimples disappear and are replaced by two prominences. If a patient has a short leg, for instance, the horizontal alignment which normally exists between the two dimples at the back will be lost. The examiner can estimate the relative heights of the two dimples by placing his thumbs on them. A difference in leg length which exceeds $1/4$ inch may indicate that the shoe has to be raised to restore the natural horizontal alignment between the two dimples. This may be a more permanent means of approaching the situation compared with manipulative treatment although the latter may be used initially. A common cause of leg shortening is an old fracture of the femur.

HISTORY

The patient is asked to describe how his present pain started. Was the onset of pain sudden or gradual? A patient may state that the pain came on while he was performing a minor task. Thus, a mother may say that she felt a sudden twinge in her back while she bent down to pick up her baby. Another patient may have felt his neck "lock" as he turned around to back up his car. A patient once stated that the felt "something like an explosion" in his back as he coughed and the pain which resulted stayed with him for 2 weeks until he was referred to the author for treatment. Sudden onset of pain is usually dramatic in nature and often followed by inability to move the affected part.

An insidious onset is less dramatic. The pain may have started as a minor ache which the patient initially ignored but which then became gradually worse until the patient was activated to seek some form of help. A man, for instance, after a day's work might have mentioned to his wife a slight ache in his lower back and asked her to rub it for him with any of the popular ointments. As the week progressed he may have noticed that it was getting worse and affecting his work until he woke up one morning to find that he could not get out of bed because the pain had not only become excruciating but was radiating to one or both of his

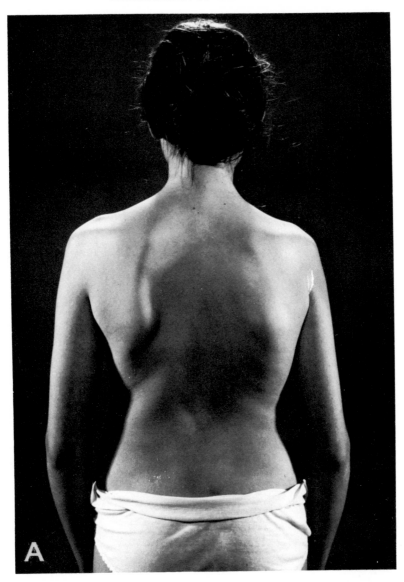

FIG. 4.1 A

FIG. 4.1. A. Posterior standing view of a subject with scoliosis. Note the thoracic lordosis. The scoliotic deformity does not seem very apparent with the patient in this position. B. The same subject shown in the forward-flexion position. A horizontal view makes the spinal deformity more apparent and reveals a right rib hump. C. An anterior-posterior roentgenogram of the subject showing a 21-degree scoliosis.

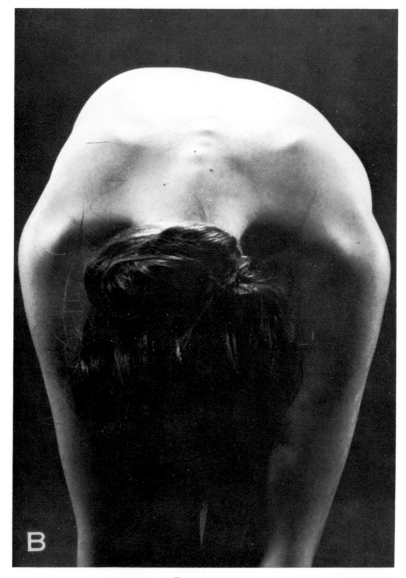

FIG. 4.1 *B*

buttocks or even his legs, and he had to call his employer to report himself sick.

Sometimes there is a history of trauma such as an automobile accident or a fall which the patient has forgotten about because there was no pain to speak of at that particular time. The present pain may be traced back to that incident. Quite often, the actual mechanism of the injury may be

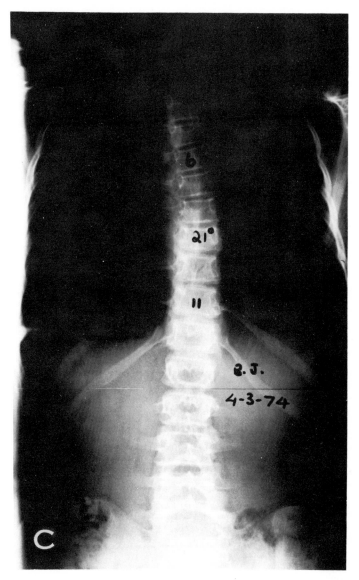

FIG. 4.1 C

important. A novice golfer might have missed the ball as he swung his trunk to the left. This might determine the kind of technique which would be effective in treating him. Lesions which have a mechanical causality are usually more amenable to manipulative therapy than those which develop spontaneously or have an insidious onset. Pains of dramatic onset can usually be eliminated in a dramatic manner.

PAIN

The patient is asked to place the tip of a finger on the exact location of his pain. Is the pain located in one spot or is it diffuse? What makes the pain better? What makes it worse? How does the pain feel first thing in the morning? How do rest and activity affect the pain? Is there any pain reference down any of the limbs? Any numbness? The distribution of referred pain and parasthesia when experienced by a patient often conforms to the dermatomes (Figure 4.2, A and B). This will help the examiner to locate the root levels involved. Pain in the region of the shoulder, for instance, will indicate a C5/C6 lesion while pain going down the front of the thigh will indicate a lesion at the L3/L4 level. Due to the overlap which exists between adjacent dermatomes, the pain distribution may act only as a guide to the level of its origin and does not always determine its exact source. Other factors such as history, spinal movements, results of palpation and position of pain must all be considered before the source of the symptoms can be located more precisely.

The patient is asked to describe the nature of his pain. Patients describe their pain in many ways—as sharp, dull, shooting, throbbing or it may be likened to a toothache. Some patients liken their pain to a situation in which "someone is driving a knife into his back." A patient once reported that his back felt as if it was "gripped in a vise."

The ability of the patient to locate the source of his pain accurately will depend on whether the source is superficial or deep. Pain of a superficial source has a sharp character to it and is easily located by the patient. When the source of pain is deep, however, it is less well localized and manifests itself as a dull and constant ache. It may be exacerbated but not suddenly by certain activities and its intensity will depend on the causative factors and severity at the source. By and large, pain of a superficial origin is felt by the patient at its point of origin whereas pain of a deep origin is felt either in the appropriate dermatome, myotome or sclerotome which has a reflex connection to the affected segment and the pain is therefore often felt at a distance away from its origin.

One other reason for poor localization of pain originating from deep structures is that dermatome and myotome areas do not correspond to each other. Gough and Koepe made electromyographic studies of erector spinae muscles of 21 subjects who had complete spinal cord injuries.[1] The results of their investigation pointed to the fact that the innervation of a ventral myotome by a spinal nerve was within two segments of the corresponding dermatome, but in the dorsal myotomes the innervation was invariably at a lower level. Based on these results, it is not surprising that in some cases there are discrepancies between the sites of pain and the lesion producing it.

Pain emanating from visceral sources such as the esophagus, kidney, gall bladder and intestinal tract may sometimes manifest itself in the back. When this occurs, spinal movements do not correlate precisely with

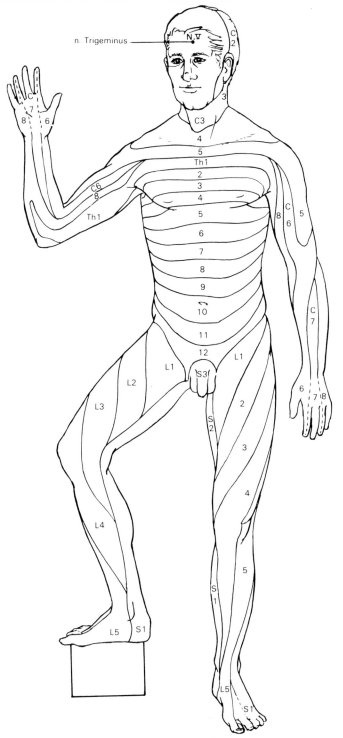

FIG. 4.2 A

FIG. 4.2. Scheme of radicular cutaneous innervations. Dermatomes.
A. Anterior view. B. Posterior view.
Reproduced from Krayenbühl, H. and Zander, E. Rupture of lumbar
and intervertebral disks. Documenta Rheumatologica Geigy No. 1,
1956, Basel. By permission of the publishers of CIBA-GEIGY Limited,
Basel, Switzerland.

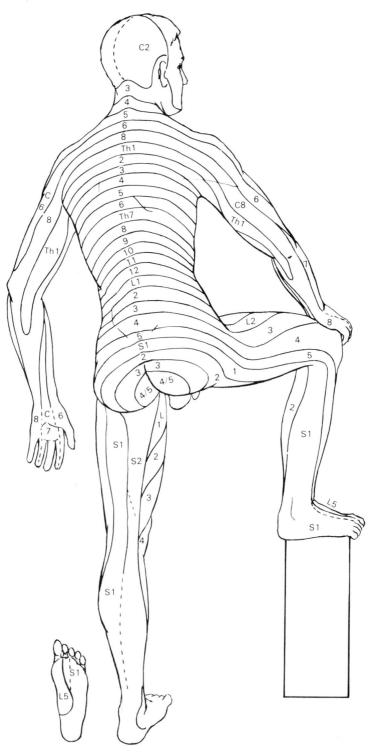

FIG. 4.2 *B*

32

the patient's distress.[2] When the patient reports that coughing hurts him in the back, more especially if it also hurts in the limbs, it may signal an interference with the dura. It should be remembered that the build-up of intra-abdominal pressure during coughing also distracts the sacroiliac joints and if a lesion is present in this region, pain may be felt in the buttock. If a patient reports that a particular posture, for example forward-bending, alleviates or exacerbates his symptoms, this points to a mechanical basis for his symptoms in that the lesion can be associated with a moving part.[3] Pain which is made worse by rest but ameliorated by activity generally responds well to manipulative therapy. Pain of a throbbing nature or nocturnal pain which is worsened by activity responds less well.

NEUROLOGICAL EXAMINATION

Neurological examination focuses attention on how much neurological deficit has resulted from the spinal lesion. In many cases it helps to predict the patient's reaction to treatment. For instance, patients who report numbness in a limb respond slowly. Neurological examination also points out those patients whose conditions might be worsened by manipulation. For example, a discovery during examination that the third and fourth sacral roots are being menaced resulting in frequency of micturition will suggest that manipulative therapy may be contraindicated.

The patient's reflexes are tested in the appropriate limbs depending on where the symptoms are emanating from. The reflexes which are usually elicited are outlined below.

Biceps reflex C5, C6 (musculocutaneous nerve), triceps reflex C6, C7 (radial nerve); upper abdominal reflex T7, T8, T9, T10; lower abdominal reflex T10, T11, T12; patellar reflex L2, L3, L4 (femoral nerve); Achilles tendon reflex S1, S2 (tibial nerve).

There is of course some overlap among adjacent levels and therefore the results should not be regarded as conclusive. It is assumed that the reader is well conversant with the methods of eliciting the above reflexes. However, in case of doubt the appropriate textbooks on neurology should be consulted.

The examiner tests the patient for sensory changes. Pin pricks can be used for this purpose. A good way to record the results is to use a body chart. This gives an on-the-glance visual record. Quite often there is no sensory loss but there may be impairment of appreciation of light touch and tactile discrimination in the limbs.

The examiner assesses the relevant limb for the presence of root paresis. Any signs of motor weakness are noted and the relevant myotome identified. For instance, weakness of the quadriceps muscle group in the lower limbs points to the affection of L2, L3 and L4 roots while weakness of the deltoid muscle in the upper limb would indicate that C5, C6 roots are affected (see Figure 4.3, A and B.)

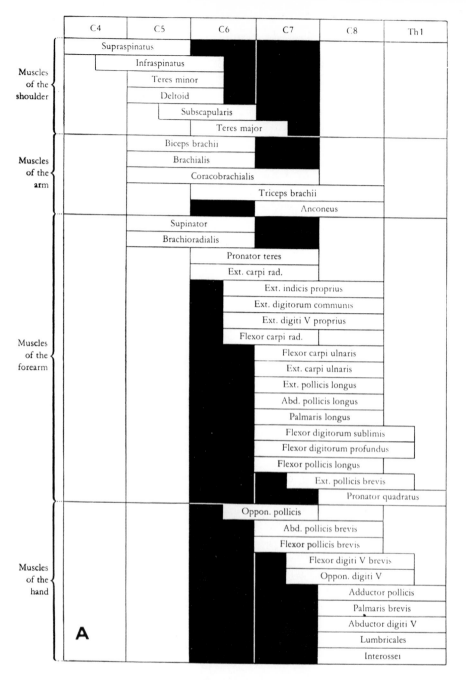

FIG. 4.3 A

FIG. 4.3. A. Segmental innervation of the muscles of the upper extremities. B. Segmental innervation of the muscles of the lower extremities.

Reproduced from Krayenbühl, H. and Zander, E. Rupture of lumbar and cervical intervertebral disks. Documenta Rheumatologica Geigy No. 1, 1956, Basel. By permission of the publishers CIBA-GEIGY Limited, Basel, Switzerland.

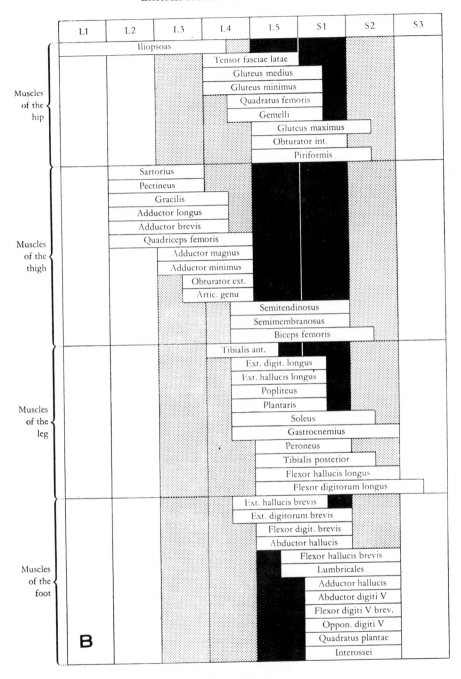

FIG. 4.3 B

Lasègue's (Straight-Leg-Raising) Test

This test is used to determine if L4, L5 and S1 nerve roots are being menaced by pressure and if so, to what extent since the result can be quantified to a useful extent. This test is conducted with the patient in the supine position with the knees in the extended position and the ankles plantarflexed. The examiner holds the patient's leg and raises it by causing flexion at the hip. If the L4, L5 and S1 roots are affected the patient will report pain which is often severe in the lower back, in the affected leg or both. The angle to which the leg can be raised invariably correlates negatively with the severity of root involvement. The angle which the leg makes with the horizontal is noted. This constitutes a useful yardstick with which the efficacy of treatment can be assessed. A patient who demonstrates a straight-leg-raising of 20 degrees pre-treatment and 40 degrees post-treatment has shown an improvement. The normal individual demonstrates a wide range of the angle of straight-leg-raising which could vary from about 65 to 120 degrees. In many cases limitation is due to tightness of the hamstrings producing an uncomfortable feeling at the back of the knee.

It should be remembered that when this test is being carried out the patient's pelvis should not be allowed to be lifted off the examination table or rotate forward since this might distort the correct picture.

Not infrequently, limitation of straight-leg-raising could be due to the presence of a sacroiliac lesion. A true positive Lasègue's sign is pain on the dorsiflexion of the foot. If the foot is dorsiflexed and no pain is produced in the back or affected leg, attention should be focused on the sacroiliac joint.

Ely's Test (Prone-Lying Knee-Flexion)

This test is utilized to determine if there is involvement of the L3, L4 roots. The patient is asked to lie prone with the hips in the extended position. The examiner attempts to flex the knee of the affected leg. This maneuver stretches the anterior aspect of the thigh. If there is limitation of flexion due to pain, it is indicative of involvement of the third and fourth lumbar nerve roots due to encroachment on the intervertebral foramen thereby placing a restriction on its mobility.

GROSS SPINAL MOVEMENTS

The patient is asked to perform active movements of the area of the spine under examination. A positive correlation invariably exists between movement limitation and severity of symptoms. The movements which are limited are recorded as is the extent of limitation. The measurement of joint limitation provides a basis from which post-treatment joint status can be assessed. If a particular movement appears to be painless, the examiner applies a gentle but firm pressure in the direction of the movement at the apparent end of the range in order to be certain that it really is painless. A particular movement, when initially viewed cursorily, may appear normal but if the patient is asked to perform the same movement repeatedly, a localized limitation within two vertebrae may come to light (Figure 4.4, A and B).

Spinal movement should be accompanied by a smooth and syncronous unfolding of the spinous processes, as during forward flexion. When the spine returns to the starting position the reverse event should take place with the spine folding up in a syncronous manner (Figure 4.5). If localized areas of rigidity are observed they should be suspected for pathology. The movements which should be tested are flexion, extension, side-flexion to both sides and rotation to both sides. Movements which show limitation and those which produce pain should be noted.

When the patient reports pain during extension and has no problems with other movements, it suggests that the facets are being compressed before the movement reaches its maximum extent. Proportionate limitation of all movements is frequently associated with degenerative conditions of the spine with contracture of the capsules of the apophyseal joints. Parasthesia, when present, is often aggravated by one or more spinal movements in cases where there is nerve root compression. Sometimes the pain which the patient complains of is unaffected by any of the spinal movements. This suggests that the pain is of non-spinal origin and may have its seat in the viscera.

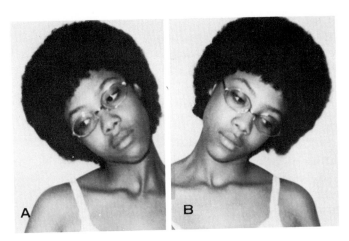

Fig. 4.4. A. Examination of side-flexion movements of the neck. At first it seemed as if both side-flexion to the left and to the right were equal. B. On examination during repeated movements, it was noticed that side-flexion to the left was limited. There was also intervertebral limitation between C3 and C4 levels.

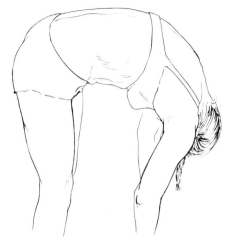

FIG. 4.5. Spinal movement accompanied by smooth and synchron-ous processes, in forward flexion.

INTERVERTEBRAL MOBILITY TESTS

The tests which have been discussed are usually sufficient to lead the examiner to the troublesome joint. Occasionally, however, the examiner may be at loss at locating the affected joint. Intervertebral mobility tests then become useful. These tests determine the degree of movement which exists in an intervertebral joint. The tests are performed by moving the section of the patient's spine under examination through a full passive range and palpating the extent of movement taking place between two spinous processes. This is then compared to that existing in the interspinous spaces lying superiorly and inferiorly. It must be noted that these movements are very small indeed and require sensitive fingers to detect them. Various tests for intervertebral mobility exist. This section will outline the techniques which can be easily and quickly performed. The tests cover the whole of the spine, with the exception of the atlanto-axial joint which is difficult to palpate.

Examination of Occipito-Atlantal Movement

(See Figure 4.6.) The patient is asked to lie down in the supine position on a table with her head resting on a pillow. The examiner places his left hand under the patient's occiput in such a way that the tip of his left thumb is lying between the mastoid process and the transverse process of the atlas. With the right hand which is gripping the patient's forehead he rotates the patient's head to the left and then to the right in a back-and-forth fashion. At the time that full rotation is being approached, the examiner will be able to feel with his left thumb that the transverse process will tend to move in the direction of the mastoid process. As the head is moved back to mid-range the transverse process will also be felt to move in a direction away from the patient's mastoid process.

Examination of Flexion (C2-C7)

(See Figure 4.7.) The patient is lying supine on the table. The operator, who is standing at the head of the table, lifts her head up with the right hand. He places his left hand on the left aspect of the patient's neck with the tip of his left thumb between the two spinous processes of the

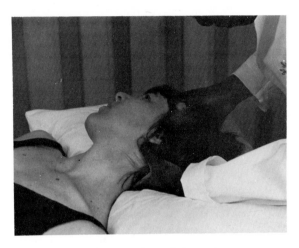

FIG. 4.6. Examination of occipito-atlantal movement.

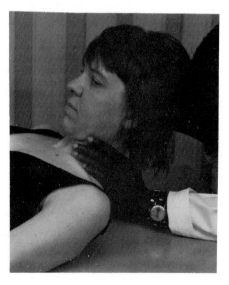

FIG. 4.7. Examination of cervical flexion (C2-C7).

vertebrae of which intervertebral movement he is examining. With the right hand the examiner flexes and extends the patient's head and neck. As these movements take place, he simultaneously palpates the intervertebral movements which are taking place between the two spinous processes. What the left thumb will feel are closing and opening movements which take place as the head is gently rocked back and forth.

Examination of Flexion (C6-T4)

(See Figure 4.8.) The patient is asked to sit down on a chair. The examiner, who is standing on her right side, places his right hand on her head with the left thumb positioned to palpate between two spinous processes. The examiner rocks the head gently back and forth while palpating with the left thumb.

Examination of Thoracic Rotation (T4-T12)

(See Figure 4.9.) The patient is in the sitting position and the examiner is standing behind her. She is asked to place her right hand behind her head. The examiner passes his right arm through the triangular space created by the patient's arm positioning so that his hand rests on the patient's cervical region. Using the available leverage, he rotates the patient's spine while simultaneously palpating for interspinous movement with the left thumb.

Examination of Lumbar Flexion (L1-L5)

(See Figure 4.10.) The patient is side-lying on her right side with flexed knees and hips. The examiner, who is standing in front of the patient, grasps the patient's knees at the posterior part. He then slightly lifts and

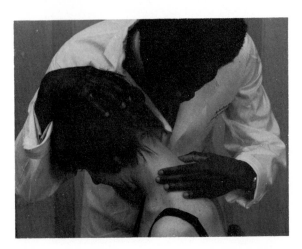

FIG. 4.8. Examination of flexion (C6-T4).

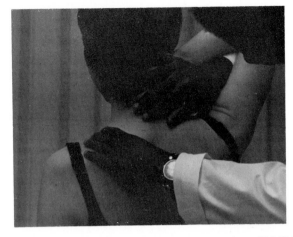

FIG. 4.9. Examination of thoracic rotation (T4-T12).

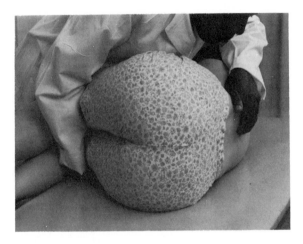

FIG. 4.10. Examination of lumbar flexion (L1-L5).

places the patient's knees firmly against his thighs. He reaches over the patient and places the tips of his fingers on the lumbar interspinous spaces to be palpated. In this starting position the examiner is able to flex the patient's lumbar spine in a rhythmic manner by repeatedly applying pressure intermittently using the right hand on the posterior aspect of the patient's knees and simultaneously applying pressure using the front part of his thighs on the patient's lower limbs. The lumbar flexion which this maneuver causes is transmitted through hip flexion. The fingers of the examiner's left hand palpate the rhythmic opening and closing taking place in the interspinous spaces.

EXAMINATION OF THE SACROILIAC JOINT

The sacroiliac joint is not directly controlled by any muscle which can be palpated for spasm. Physical examination depends on palpation for tenderness in the region of the joint itself and testing for lack of mobility.

Not infrequently when no positive results are obtained after treatment of the lumbar region, the source of the pain may be found in the sacroiliac region. However, evaluation of the degree of mobility in the sacroiliac joint requires sensitive fingers since the movement which takes place in this joint is very small indeed. Quite often when there is a lesion in the sacroiliac joint, the patient reports tenderness in the region medial to the posterior inferior iliac spine.

Horizontal Compression Test

(See Figure 4.11.) The patient is asked to lie supine on the table. The examiner who is standing on her right side applies pressure with both hands on the patient's ilia. The direction of both pressures is toward the mid-line. This maneuver produces a gapping effect on the sacroiliac joints. If the patient finds this test painful, it may point to pathology in the sacroiliac joints.

Vertical Compression Test

(See Figure 4.12.) The patient is supine-lying. The examiner stands on her right side and places both hands on the anterior superior iliac spines. From this position the examiner applies a gentle but firm downward pressure slightly laterally. This maneuver stretches the anterior sacroiliac ligament especially. The procedure constitutes a sensitive test for detecting pathology in the sacroiliac joints. If the patient reports pain in the sacroiliac region pathology should be suspected.

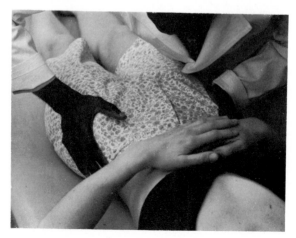

FIG. 4.11. Horizontal compression test on the sacroiliac joints.

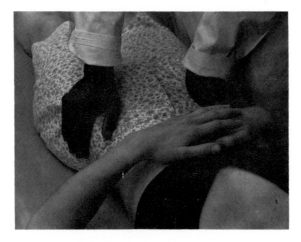

FIG. 4.12. Vertical compression test on the sacroiliac joints.

GENERAL CONSIDERATION AND OTHER TESTS

End-Feel

When the examiner puts a joint through the available range, the type of resistance which he encounters at the terminal stage of the range varies. This resistance is designated in manipulative jargon by the term, "end-feel." Sometimes the resistance comes on like a sudden block immediately putting a stop to any further passive movement. When this kind of end-feel is accompanied by severe muscle spasm, the use of manipulative therapy may be contraindicated although this may not exclude the gentler techniques. Sometimes the end-feel can be likened to a "spongy" resistance with considerable give and sometimes there is a hard spongy opposition at the end of the available range. This is often encountered among middle-aged patients with degenerative changes in the spine including capsular contracture.

Vertical Compression on Spinous Processes

This procedure is done by the application of direct vertical pressure on the spinous processes of the suspected vertebral levels, using the thumb. Pain is invariably elicited from vertebral levels which are causing symptoms. The examiner should proceed gently with this test because in cases where the condition is acute, it could be a very painful procedure for the patient.

Testing Thoracic Resilience

(See Figure 4.13.) The patient is lying prone on the table with the examiner standing on her left side. The examiner now places his right hand on the patient's thoracic region with the pisiform bone on the spinous process. From this position the examiner applies a vertical pressure on the back. This is applied in a rhythmic manner to the levels the examiner wishes to assess. This test gives the examiner an idea as to the "springiness" or resilience in the thoracic spine or stiffness in the back, if present.

Skin-Rolling Test

(See Figure 4.14.) This test involves lifting the skin by the forefingers and the thumbs and rolling and gently squeezing it over the spinous processes of the area of the spine under examination. Invariably, the patient will report tenderness which will be maximal over the vertebral

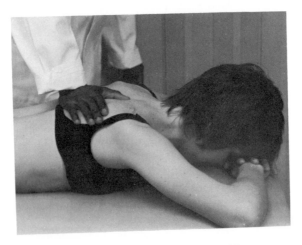

FIG. 4.13. Testing thoracic resilience.

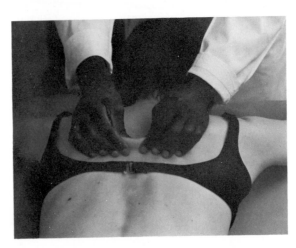

FIG. 4.14. Skin-rolling test.

level in which the joint lesion exists. When performing this test it should be remembered that in some patients there is natural tenderness in the thoracic region and this may mislead the examiner.

Hip-Rolling Test

The examiner uses this test to find out if there is pathology in the hip which sometimes might obfuscate the clinical picture when the hip is being moved during examination of the back. The test is easily done while the patient is lying supine. It involves rolling the outstretched leg back and forth thus causing outward and inward rotation of the hip.

The Radiologist's Report

It is usually expedient to read the radiologist's report. The importance of an X-ray picture of the spine lies in the fact that it is a screening device. It helps the referring physician to exclude those patients whose X-rays have indicated serious disease processes which would contraindicate manipulative treatment. Kraus makes the point, however, that organic disease makes up only a small percentage of back pain.[4] Some of the diseases which may manifest themselves as back pain and which can be detected by an X-ray examination are Paget's disease, osteoporosis, metastases, osteomyelitis and spondylolisthesis.

One of the striking features of spinal X-rays is that they do not show a consistent correlation with the patient's symptoms. As a result, the radiological picture may indicate gross degenerative changes whereas the patient's symptoms may be mild in comparison, with the patient reporting only occasional minor twinges. On the other hand, a patient whose X-ray shows relatively unpronounced degenerative changes may report gross symptoms. Of course, sometimes the X-ray impression matches the symptoms but the point here is that the situation does not follow any hard and fast rules. In addition, symptoms of radicular pain do not always correspond to the root level affected by the foraminal deformity.[5]

Straight X-rays do not show joint hypermobility, strain of the apophyseal joints and spinal positional faults. However, they help to give the examiner a good impression about the bony condition of the spinal area under consideration, thus adding depth to the general clinical picture which the examiner is trying to form.[6] If the radiologist's report, for instance, indicates that a patient's spine demonstrates osteoporotic changes, this will caution the examiner as to how much pressure he can apply while administering a manipulative technique after examination.

REFERENCES

1. Gough, J. G. and Koepe, G. H. E. M. G. Determination of motor root levels in erector spinae muscles. Arch. Phys. Med., 47: 9, 1966.

2. Ferguson, R. H. *Medical Evaluation of Backache and Neckache* (Gurdjian, C. and Thomas, C. M., Eds.) Charles C Thomas, Springfield, Illinois, 1970.
3. Cyriax, J. *Textbook of Orthopaedic Medicine*, vol. I. Cassell, London, 1965.
4. Kraus, H. *Backache, Stress and Tension: Their Care, Prevention and Treatment*. Simon and Schuster, New York, 1965.
5. Stoddard, A. Manipulation for low backache. Rheumatism, *16:* 20–24, 1960.
6. Paris, S. V. *Spinal Lesion*. Pegasus Press, Christchurch, New Zealand, 1965.

Chapter 5

Techniques of spinal manipulation

In the practice of manipulative therapy there are scores of techniques available to the manipulative therapist. There is also a limitless number of modifications of the "core techniques" and improvisations which can be created to suit each case. Some of these techniques are simple to perform, some difficult, and some are flamboyant and impressive to the onlooker. Most of the techniques employed by practitioners have either osteopathic or chiropractic components although some occasionally make use of Cyriax' and Mennell's techniques.

Over the years there have been extensive borrowing and absorption of techniques among the various schools.[1] The resulting hybridization has led to the loss of the origins of many of the techniques used today in clinical practice. Despite this situation it is still possible to find certain broad differences between osteopathic and chiropractic approaches to manipulation. Most chiropractors employ direct thrusts which cause extension of the intervertebral joint under manipulation and it is important to them that a click accompanies the manipulation. In chiropractic thinking this supposedly means that the joint has been clicked back into place and normal alignment restored. A considerable degree of force characterizes chiropractic manipulations. On the other hand specificity and gentleness characterize osteopathic techniques. The osteopath only employs the more powerful techniques when the gentler ones have not done the job.[2] The great advantage of the gentler techniques which are described as "articulatory" techniques is their ease of application combined with ease of acquiring application skill for those with the necessary aptitude. The techniques can be used in the presence of disease if applied within the limits of pain. Stoddard has outlined osteopathic techniques in an excellent manner in his book.[3] The reader who desires more information on the subject will find his publication interesting.

By and large manipulative techniques can be classified under the headings indirect manipulations, direct manipulations, specific manipulations, non-specific manipulations, oscillatory techniques, and manipulative thrusts.

Indirect Manipulations

When using these techniques the operator utilizes the limbs as natural levers to influence the spinal column. For example, when a patient is side-lying with the operator applying pressure on the pelvis and the shoulder in opposite directions, the resulting force can cause torsion of the lumbar spine.

Direct Manipulations

These involve direct manual pressure on the vertebrae in order to influence the intervertebral joints under treatment. Direct manipulations are sometimes described as pressure techniques.

Specific Manipulations

These are manipulative techniques intended to influence only one joint at a time. This purpose is achieved in several ways.

Positioning of the Area of Spine under Treatment

When treating the cervical spine, for instance, the operator should position the neck in the mid-position between flexion and extension before the manipulative force can fall on the mid-cervical intervertebral joints. When manipulation of the cervical spine is attempted with the head and neck in flexion or extension at the level of the upper cervical spine, the manipulative force falls between the first cervical vertebra and the occiput. If the head is in the extended position and manipulation is administered with the neck in rotation and side-flexion to the opposite side it is the joint between the first and second cervical vertebrae which is affected. However, when the upper cervical spine is manipulated with the neck in rotation and side-flexion to the same side most of the manipulative force falls on the joint between the second and third cervical vertebrae. This is because when rotation and side-flexion occur to the same side the joint between the first and second vertebrae becomes blocked. When manipulation of the upper lumbar intervertebral joints is desired the lumbar spine should be placed in extension. The lower lumbar intervertebral joints would need a flexed spine.

Locking

The architectural design of the facets is such that rotation follows side-flexion of the spine. The prevention of that rotatory component will force the facets against each other, precipitating a state known as "facet apposition locking" in manipulative jargon. This mechanical principle is utilized in localizing forces during manipulation of the spine and it is also a device which helps to protect the joints below and above the vertebral level under consideration so that they are not traumatized. The other method used to effect locking is ligamentous tension, achieved by moving the joint to the limit of joint range possible and utilizing the resulting capsular tension to lock the joint.

Leverage of Movement

This is another way to achieve specificity. For instance, it is possible to localize the manipulative force in the lumbar spine by utilizing the leverage of movement from above or below. Following this principle, the trunk can be rotated on a relatively fixed spine for the treatment of the upper lumbar intervertebral joints. The treatment of lower lumbar intervertebral joints can be effected by rotating the pelvis on a relatively fixed trunk. To localize the manipulative force to the intervertebral joints in the mid-lumbar region the operator has to coordinate pelvic and trunk rotations appropriately; usually the pelvic and trunk rotations have to be proportionately equal to each other.

Non-Specific Manipulations

These are techniques whereby the manipulative force falls on more than one joint. Most of Cyriax' techniques fall under this category in which massive traction is applied to the area of the spine under treatment simultaneously with the manipulative thrust.[4]

Oscillatory Techniques

These techniques could be described as gentle forms of manipulation. The oscillations can either involve rotation or pressure-release sequence.

Those that involve pressure are usually specific to one intervertebral joint whereas those that involve rotation may or may not be so. The important point about these techniques is that the operator oscillates into the patient's pain but not beyond it. The rate of oscillation—depending on which part of the spine is being treated, the operator, and pain intensity—will vary between 120 to 160 times per minute. Another important feature of these techniques is that the patient is the controller of the treatment and the possibility of hurting him is minimized. This is because the patient is constantly informing the operator whether or not the treatment is still within a tolerable level, which guides the operator with regard to the depth of the oscillations. Apart from gentleness and oscillations, the other component of these techniques is rhythmicity. The more rhythmic the oscillations, the more tolerable and pleasant the treatment will be for the patient and the more effective. The point has to be made that gentleness has to be interpreted through the patient's perception and not through the operator's.

More than anyone else, Maitland has successfully evolved an excellent system for the application of oscillatory techniques.[1, 5] The procedures he outlined have a heavy osteopathic coloring. In the application of oscillatory techniques the operator is guided by the signs and symptoms which the patient brings into the treatment situation. The fact that the patient may have a lumbar disc lesion, facet lesion, spondylosis, Schmorl's modes or any diagnostic label is de-emphasized. Moreover, the operator attempts to increase the existing amount of movement in the joint which is the subject of treatment. This purpose is very much facilitated if the joint is positioned somewhere in mid-range relative to all of its other ranges when the operator wishes to move the joint in a chosen direction. With this principle in mind, in order to treat the mid-cervical region with rotation, the neck should be flexed to an angle whereby the mid-cervical region lies mid-way between flexion and extension. If rotation of the upper lumbar region is desired, the lumbar region should be positioned in extension; the lower lumbar region requires flexion. The use of oscillatory pressure requires that the pressure should be directed at 90 degrees to the vertebral spinous process in order to achieve maximal effect.

Manipulative Thrusts

The techniques classified under this heading represent a more powerful approach to joint movement. They are characterized by high velocity movements although the amplitudes are small. The manipulative thrust takes place so fast that it beats the reaction time of the patient. This situation therefore is potentially dangerous in that the patient loses the ability to control the treatment, in contrast to oscillatory techniques.

The point has to be made that the above classifications are for descriptive purposes only. For practical purposes in clinical practice such compartmentalization is not possible. As a result any chosen technique may be impregnated with one or more of the elements described above. For example a chosen technique may be oscillatory in nature and it may be specific or non-specific. Another technique may be a manipulative thrust; at the same time it may be indirect or direct. It may be specific or non-specific.

The rest of this chapter will attempt to outline the manipulative techniques which the author has found to be the most efficacious in his own practice. The postures of patient and operator which will be described are for guidance only. They can be modified as long as one does not lose sight of the basic principles. The technique will cover the cervical, thoracic and lumbar regions, followed by techniques for the sacroiliac joints.

Vertical Oscillatory Pressure, Cervical Region

(See Figure 5.1.) The patient is asked to lie prone with her head resting on the back of her hands. Standing at the head end of the table, the operator places the pads of his thumbs on the spinous process of the vertebra to be manipulated. His fingers are spread out on the sides of the patient's neck.

Vertical oscillatory pressure is executed by the rhythmic application of pressure on the spinous process followed by relaxation. The origin of the pressure is from the operator's trunk flexion; the origin of the relaxation is from trunk extension. The operator's shoulders and elbows are held in flexion and extension, respectively. His arms act as rigid pillars through which the trunk movements are transmitted to the thumbs and then to the spinous process. Application of pressure by the contraction of the intrinsics of the hands should be avoided.

When applied in the neck region vertical oscillatory techniques are

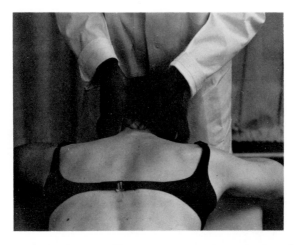

FIG. 5.1. Vertical oscillatory pressure, cervical region.

highly versatile. They are, however, particularly useful when the patient states that his pain has a bilateral distribution in relation to the mid-line of the back of the neck. It does not seem to matter whether the pain is localized to the cervical region itself or is referred bilaterally to the upper limbs and head. These techniques also seem to produce better results when the patient has reached middle age or when the radiologist's report indicates signs of degeneration in the cervical region.

Some patients complain of lassitude and languor, some complain of being sick, and some have reported that they vomitted 20 to 30 minutes after treatment. It is, therefore, good practice to mention the possibility of these side effects to the patient to stave off any feeling of alarm, especially if the upper cervical vertebrae have been manipulated or if it has been necessary to use great depth of pressure when using this technique. These post-treatment side effects are temporary and should not be cause for concern.

Transverse Oscillatory Pressure, Cervical Region

(See Figure 5.2.) The patient is asked to lie prone on the table with her forehead placed on the backs of her fingers. Standing on the left side of the patient, the operator places the pads of his thumbs against the left side of the spinous process of the vertebrae to be moved. His fingers are spread out on the neck and upper thoracic region.

Pressure is directed horizontally through the thumbs to the side of the spinous process. Transverse oscillatory pressure is executed by a pressure-relax sequence on the spinous process. Movement is initiated from the trunk, and transmitted down the arms to the thumbs.

This technique is useful when pain has a unilateral distribution, whether localized to the neck or referred to the upper limb. When this

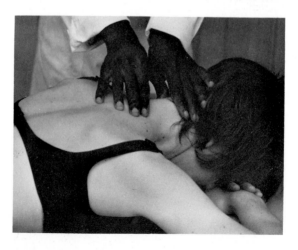

FIG. 5.2. Transverse oscillatory pressure, cervical region.

technique is applied, therapeutic effect is maximized if pressure is applied toward the side of the patient's pain. In Figure 5.2 it is assumed that the patient's pain is located on her right side.

Oscillatory Rotation, Cervical Region

(See Figure 5.3.) The patient is asked to lie supine with her head extending beyond the head end of the table. The operator, who is standing at the head end of the table, supports the patient's head by grasping her occiput with his left hand. He places his right hand on her chin. He moves close to the patient and gives her head additional support using his right elbow and abdomen.

Oscillatory rotation to the cervical region is administered by gradually turning the head and neck to the right side, using both hands and then derotating in an oscillatory manner. The derotation which goes in the left direction commences when the rotation just elicits pain or muscle spasm. Both hands should be working together in close partnership to produce this rhythmic rotation-derotation oscillatory sequence.

When applied to the cervical region oscillatory rotation is useful when the patient exhibits unilateral pain distribution. The pain may be localized to the neck area or referred to the head or limbs. This technique is maximally effective when the head and neck are turned away from the pain. In Figure 5.3 it is assumed that the patient's pain is situated on her left side.

Positioning of the head and neck can be used to localize the effect of oscillatory rotation to chosen areas of the cervical spine. When the upper part of the cervical spine is under treatment, the head and neck should be positioned in the same plane with the body. To treat the intervertebral

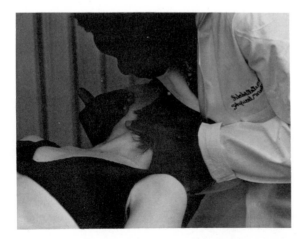

FIG. 5.3. Oscillatory rotation, cervical region. Cervical rotatory thrust.

joints of the lower cervical spine, the head and neck should be placed in flexion.

When examination has revealed that the patient suffers from dizziness or when the treatment itself causes dizziness, great caution should be entertained in the application of this procedure. If it is going to be used, an exploratory oscillatory rotation should be carried out, the patient's reaction watched, and the wisdom of doing the real treatment questioned.

Cervical Rotatory Thrust

(See Figure 5.3.) The positions adopted by the operator and patient are identical to those for cervical oscillatory rotation. The operator rotates the patient's head and neck to the right, taking up the slack. When the head and neck have reached the limit of the available range, this is followed up with a sudden high velocity, low amplitude movement.

Occipito-Atlantal Manipulation

(See Figure 5.4.) The patient is asked to lie supine on the table with her head resting on a pillow. The operator, standing at the head end of the table, places his left hand under the patient's occiput and his right hand on her chin. His left thumb is placed on the left transverse process of the atlas. The occipito-atlantal joint is stretched by rotating the head and neck to the right.

Occipito-atlantal manipulation is effected by sudden rotation of the head and neck using the right hand after taking up the slack. The left thumb functions to stop any movement of the atlas.

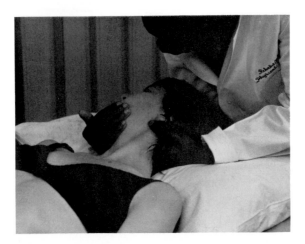

FIG. 5.4. Occipito-atlantal manipulation.

Atlanto-Axial Manipulation

(See Figure 5.5.) The patient is lying supine with her head on a pillow. The operator, standing at the head end of the table, places his left hand under her occiput and his right hand on her chin. With his right hand the operator rotates the patient's head and neck to the right to the limit of the available range.

Atlanto-axial manipulation is administered by making a short and sharp rotatory thrust. The efficacy of this technique depends on relaxation of the patient, suddenness of the maneuver, placing the neck in the mid-position, and fixing the transverse process of the axis with the left thumb for specificity. In this way the skull and atlas will act as one block in relation to the axis.

Cervical Manipulation C2-C7

(See Figure 5.6.) The patient is asked to lie supine with her head and neck extending beyond the table. The operator, standing at the head end of the table slightly to the left of the patient, supports her head with his left hand and places his right hand on her chin. The operator moves closer to the patient and increases the head support with his right elbow, right forearm and right pectoral area. His left hand is adjusted so that the radial aspect of his left index finger lies on the articular process of the two vertebrae superior to the intervertebral joint which he wishes to manipulate, making it possible for the force of the manipulation to fall on the desired intervertebral joint. The cervical region is side-flexed to the left and rotated to the right.

The cervical manipulation is administered by a rotatory thrust of high velocity and low amplitude with the right hand. This is done after all

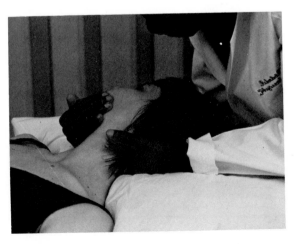

FIG. 5.5. Atlanto-axial manipulation.

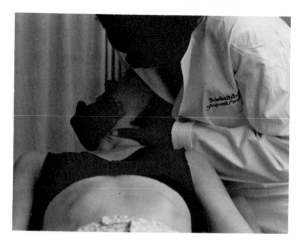

FIG. 5.6. Cervical manipulation (C2-C7).

slack has been taken up and tension is felt at the intervertebral joint which is being manipulated. The detector of the tension is the left index finger. The direction of the manipulative thrust should be upward and forward consistent with the plane of the articular facets.

This technique is a locking technique in which the operator makes use of facet locking and ligamentous tension locking. When the operator side-flexes the neck to the left he causes the left row of facets to "lock" and opens up the right row of facets. Rotation of the neck to the right causes a tightening of ligaments, specifically the capsule of the intervertebral joint to be manipulated. The manipulation itself will stretch the facet joint which lies opposite the fulcrum of movement.

Vertical Oscillatory Pressure, Thoracic Region

(See Figure 5.7.) The patient is asked to lie prone with her forehead resting on the back of her hands. Figure 5.7 shows the manipulation of the upper thoracic region. The posture of the operator and the position of the patient are identical to those described for applying vertical oscilla-tory pressure to the cervical region (Figure 5.1). When the operator desires to manipulate the mid-thoracic and lower thoracic areas he will stand on the side of the patient. He will place his thumbs in a longitudi-nal fashion on the spinous process of the vertebra to be moved. In this way his thumbs will point to each other along the spine.

Vertical oscillatory pressure is administered by a rhythmic pressure-release sequence on the spinous process using the thumbs. The pressure source is the operator's trunk with the pressure transmitted down his arms to his thumbs.

The indication for this technique for the thoracic region is when the patient's symptoms have a bilateral distribution in relation to the mid-line or when the pain is localized to the vertebral level which is being mobilized. It is also useful for symptoms which have a unilateral distribution. It is assumed of course that the patient's symptoms have a thoracic origin.

Vertical oscillatory pressure as described for the mid-thoracic and lower thoracic regions is also applicable to the lumbar spine (Figure 5.8).

Transverse Oscillatory Pressure, Thoracic Region

(See Figure 5.9.) The patient is lying prone. The operator, standing on the patient's left side, places his thumbs on the left side of the spinous

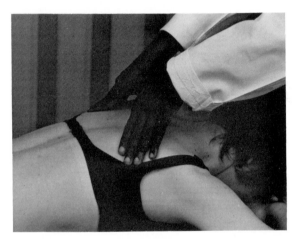

FIG. 5.7. Vertical oscillatory pressure, upper thoracic region.

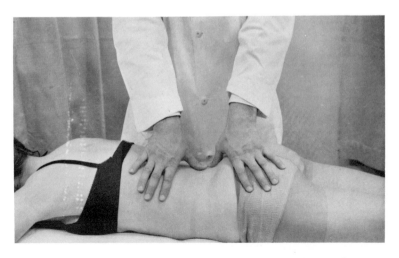

FIG. 5.8. Vertical oscillating pressure, lumbar spine.

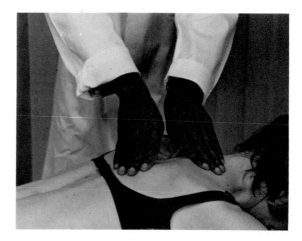

FIG. 5.9. Transverse oscillatory pressure, thoracic region.

process of the vertebra to be moved. His hands are spread out and help to stabilize his thumbs.

Transverse oscillatory pressure is administered by a push-relax sequence on the spinous process using the thumbs to produce an oscillatory movement. The thumb acts as an intermediary between the spinous process and the arms and trunk.

When it is necessary during treatment to use great pressure the patient's body will tend to roll forward with the operator's thumb pressure and then roll back. The operator's thumb pressure should be timed to coincide with the recovery phase of the patient's body. In this way the technique will tend to be in tune with the natural frequency of the patient's body. This exercise can be likened to the application of the appropriate amount of force at the recovery phase of a swinging pendulum.

Transverse oscillatory pressure to the thoracic spine is used when the patient's pain has a unilateral distribution in relation to the mid-line and is of thoracic origin. Maximal benefit is derived if the pressure is applied toward the side of the patient's pain. In this way it would seem as if the operator is rotating the vertebral body away from the pain source. Not infrequently it is necessary to apply oscillatory pressure to the adjacent costo-vertebral joints as an adjunct using the technique of vertical oscillatory pressure. The pressure is directed through the angle of the rib.

The posture of the operator and the position described above are also applicable to the treatment of the lumbar spine.

Upper Thoracic Manipulation

(See Figure 5.10.) The patient is asked to sit on a stool. The operator standing behind moves slightly to the right side of the patient. He asks

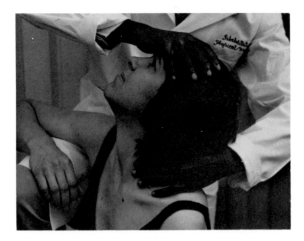

FIG. 5.10. Upper thoracic manipulation.

the patient to put her right arm on his right thigh. His right foot is placed on the stool adjacent to the patient's right buttock. The operator positions his left thumb on the left side of the spinous process of the vertebra which lies immediately below the intervertebral joint which he desires to manipulate. With his right hand grasping the patient's forehead, he puts the neck into extension, side-flexes it to the left and rotates it to the right. He can feel the tension which these neck positions cause with his left thumb.

The manipulative thrust is effected by two countermovements. One movement is with the right hand which increases neck side-flexion to the left and extension. The other movement is with the left thumb which pushes the spinous process transversely across the back. These two movements are performed simultaneously.

The use of this technique involves locking. By side-flexing the neck to the left, the operator locks this side by facet apposition. The right side which is put on stretch is fixed by ligamentous tension locking.

It has to be remembered that the upper thoracic spine is particularly difficult to manipulate. Therefore, it can not be overemphasized that any technique performed in this area should be done accurately to maximize its therapeutic value.

Vertical Thrust, Mid-Thoracic and Lower Thoracic Regions

(See Figure 5.11.) The patient is asked to lie prone on the table. The operator stands on the patient's left side and places the distal phalanges of his index and middle fingers on the transverse processes of the vertebra to be moved. This should be the vertebra below the intervertebral joint which the operator wishes to manipulate. If he desires to manipulate the intervertebral joint between T7 and T8, he should place the distal phalanges of his fingers over the transverse processes of the eighth

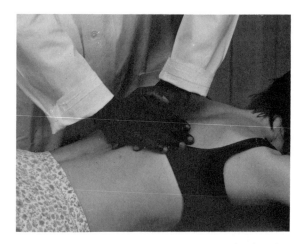

FIG. 5.11. Vertical thrust, mid-thoracic and lower thoracic regions.

thoracic vertebra. Then he places the ulnar border of his right hand over the parts of the fingers which are on the vertebral transverse processes.

The manipulative thrust is administered by a vertical force with the right hand. The force originates from the trunk and is transmitted through the right arm and right hand. The manipulation is timed to coincide with the end of the patient's expiratory phase of breathing.

Proper administration of this technique requires that the operator take note of the natural placement of the articular facets at the middle and lower thoracic areas. As a result, the manipulative thrust should go toward a caudal direction when he is treating the mid-thoracic areas, and in a cephalic direction with the lower thoracic region.

Lumbar Oscillatory Rotation

(See Figure 5.12.) The patient is asked to lie on her left side. The operator is standing behind her. He flexes the patient's right lower limb at the hip and knee and pulls on her left arm as if toward the ceiling thus rotating her trunk toward the right until it is almost eliciting pain. Her left lower limb is kept straight. The operator places his right hand on the patient's right buttock and his left hand on her right shoulder area.

Oscillatory rotation is effected with his right hand on the patient's buttock in a push-relax sequence. His left hand functions to stabilize her thorax by holding onto her left shoulder.

During oscillatory rotation, especially when a strong force is required, the patient's body will roll back and forth. The "push" component of this technique should be imparted immediately at the end of the recovery phase of the patient's rolling so that the technique is in tune with the oscillating frequency of the patient's body.

A measure of localization can be achieved by the degree of hip-flexion

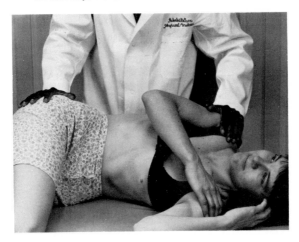

FIG. 5.12. Lumbar oscillatory rotation.

and the way in which the manipulative force is imparted on the buttock. Placement of the hand should be in the neighborhood of the iliac crest if it is desired to rotate the lumbar spine in extension. If the lumbar spine is to be rotated in flexion the right hand should be placed near the greater trochanter of the right femur. The more the right hip is flexed, the more lumbar-flexion there will be. When this is the case the manipulative force will tend to fall more on the lower lumbar spine. As the spine is moved toward extension it is the intervertebral joints in the middle and upper lumbar regions which receive the manipulative impact.

Lumbar oscillatory rotation is used when the patient's pain has a unilateral distribution and when it is localized on one side of the back in relation to the mid-line or radiating to the buttock or lower limb. To derive maximal benefit from this technique, it is administered with the patient lying on the non-painful side. In this way the pelvis is being rotated away from the side of the pain. In Figure 5.12 it is assumed that the patient's pain is situated on her right side.

Vertical Thrust, Lumbar Region

(See Figure 5.13.) The patient is prone-lying with the operator standing on her left side. The operator places the ulnar border of his right hand on the patient's back so that the pisiform bone lies on the spinous process of the vertebra which he intends to move. He tucks the small, ring and middle fingers of his left hand under the palm of his right hand between the right thumb and index finger. His left thumb and index finger are lying on the back of his right hand. In this way the left hand reinforces as it grasps the right hand.

Vertical thrust is delivered by the right hand after taking up the necessary slack. The manipulative force comes from the trunk and is transmitted down the arms to the right hand.

Lumbar Rotation, "Pump-Handle" Technique

(See Figure 5.14.) The patient is asked to lie supine. The operator stands on her right side. Placing his left hand on the patient's left shoulder he grasps the patient's right lower limb at the back of the knee with his right hand, flexing the left hip and knee to a right angle. Using the left knee as a handle he adducts the left hip and brings the left knee across the body. In the process the lumbar spine is put into rotation.

The manipulation is executed by pulling the knee toward the floor. The

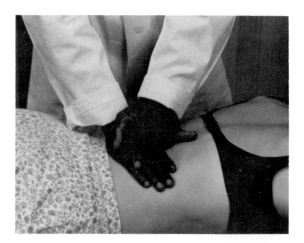

Fig. 5.13. Vertical thrust, lumbar region.

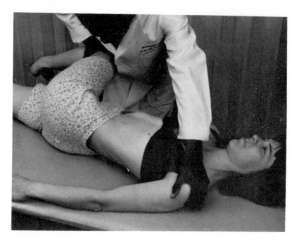

Fig. 5.14. Lumbar rotation, "pump-handle" technique.

left hand functions to hold down the left shoulder thereby indirectly holding down the thorax.

A measure of localization can be achieved by placing the lumbar spine in flexion or extension. This can be done by positioning the right leg and changing the angle of hip-flexion. More hip-flexion produces more lumbar spine-flexion, and more tendency for the manipulative thrust to fall on the lower lumbar intervertebral joints. The reverse is the case as the hip goes into extension.

Elderly patients should be treated with caution with this technique because of the unreliability of the neck of femur and the amount of torque on the hip joint due to the long leverage being used.

Specific Lumbar Rotation

(See Figure 5.15.) The patient lies on her right side. The operator stands facing her. He leans forward and passes his left arm through the space provided by the patient's left arm which is flexed at the elbow. The operator flexes the patient's left hip with his right hand using the knee to a point whereby this causes flexion at the lumbar region, specifically at the vertebral level which the operator wishes to manipulate. His left hand is used to detect this. When it happens the flexed leg is held in position by the operator's right thigh. The operator rotates the patient's trunk to the right by pulling her right arm toward the ceiling. The rotation is continued until the trunk is rotated down to the intervertebral joint to be manipulated. With his right forearm on the patient's left buttock, he places his right index finger on the right side of the spinous process of the lumbar vertebrae below the intervertebral joint to be manipulated. His left thumb is placed against the left side of the spinous

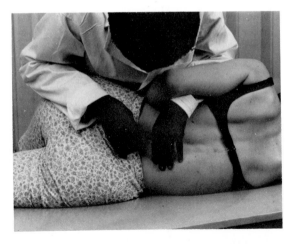

FIG. 5.15. Specific lumbar rotation.

process of the vertebrae above the intervertebral joint under manipulation.

Manipulation is executed by thrusting with the left thumb in a downward direction while the left index finger applies an upward thrust. These two counterthrusts may be augmented simultaneously by pressure on the patient's left buttock using the right forearm.

It has to be mentioned that this is a somewhat difficult technique to perform. To become proficient at it requires some practice.

Vertical Thrust, Sacroiliac Joint

(See Figure 5.16.) The patient is asked to lie prone on the table. The operator, standing on her left side, places his right hand in such a way that it lies across the right iliac crest. His left hand is positioned along the apex of the sacrum.

The operator implements the manipulative thrust by applying a vertical thrust using both hands, causing a torsion of the sacroiliac joint.

The application of torsion in the opposite direction requires that the operator place one hand on the base of the sacrum and the other on the ischial tuberosity.

Vertical thrust is a useful technique when the patient's pain is localized to the sacroiliac region or is radiating to the lower limb, or if pain is exacerbated by bending forward or sitting down, or in some cases of postpartum sacroiliac strain. Provided that the origin of the pain is in the sacroiliac joint and the nature of the pain fits into the above pattern, this is the first choice of technique. If the expected result is not realized, torsion in the opposite direction should be applied. In Figure 5.16 the manipulative thrust is being applied to the right sacroiliac joint.

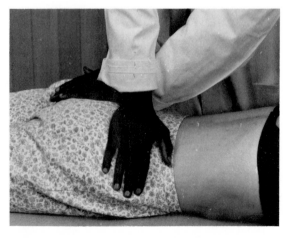

FIG. 5.16. Vertical thrust, sacroiliac joint.

Rotatory Thrust, Sacroiliac Joint

(See Figure 5.17.) The patient is asked to lie supine. Standing on her right side, the operator flexes the patient's right hip and knee maximally and places his chin on the patient's right knee to maintain the position of the fully flexed hip. He tucks his right hand under the patient's right buttock and grasps the ischial tuberosity. His left hand is placed in the anterior iliac crest area.

The rotatory thrust is administered by exerting a rotatory force with the right hand. The left hand is holding onto the right iliac crest. This technique involves pivoting the ilium on the sacrum. The direction of the manipulative force is cephalic and upward. It is the second and third sacral levels that receive most of the rotatory force.

This technique is particularly useful when the patient says that her symptoms are often relieved when she sits down and elevates her feet to a higher level than her hips. If the pain is of sacroiliac origin this should be the first choice of manipulative treatment. It does not matter whether the pain is localized in the sacroiliac region or radiating to the lower limb. In Figure 5.17 it is assumed that the symptoms are emanating from the right sacroiliac joint.

Counterclockwise Rotation, Sacroiliac Joint

(See Figure 5.18.) The patient is asked to lie on her left side. The operator is standing behind her. He flexes her right hip and knee and places her right leg in front of her left leg. He grasps the patient's left arm and pulls it toward the ceiling thus rotating the trunk to the limit and locking the spine. The patient's right leg should rest over the side of the table, causing some gapping strain on the posterior aspect of the sacroiliac joint. The operator places his right hand on the patient's right

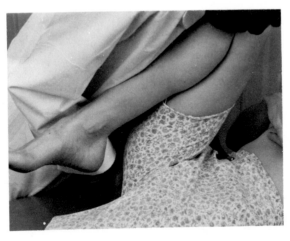

FIG. 5.17. Rotatory thrust, sacroiliac joint.

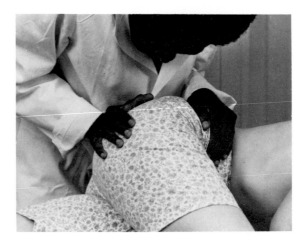

FIG. 5.18. Counterclockwise rotation, sacroiliac joint.

ischial tuberosity. His left hand is on the patient's right anterior superior iliac spine.

The counterclockwise manipulation is effected by a low amplitude high velocity thrust on the patient's ischial tuberosity. This is simultaneously coordinated with the same type of movement by the left hand. While the right hand is pushing away from the operator, the left hand is pushing toward him.

When using this technique the operator must remember that a large amount of thrusting force is required to obtain the desired effect, because he is operating with small lever arms. He should not lose sight of the fact that the amplitude of the thrust should be small.

This technique can be used as a mechanical readjustment of the sacroiliac joint, if, for instance examination revealed that the patient's symptoms were a result of subjecting the sacroiliac joint to clockwise strain, as in the case of a dentist who had strained his sacroiliac joint by twisting and turning during his work, or as in the case of a neophyte golfer who took a shot in the wrong way or missed the ball. Pain is usually exacerbated by simulating the movement which precipitated the condition. The history has to be studied and treatment applied accordingly. This technique also shares the indication of rotatory thrust for sacroiliac joint (Figure 5.17).

REFERENCES

1. Winer, C. E. R. Training in manual therapy: The current situation. Med. J. Aust., 2: 937–940, 1974.
2. Stoddard, A. Osteopathic techniques of manipulation. Physiotherapy, 56: 29–30, 1970.
3. Stoddard, A. Outline of Osteopathic Technique. Hutchinson, London, 1969.
4. Cyriax, J. Textbook of Orthopaedic Medicine, vol. II. Cassell, London, 1965.
5. Maitland, G. Vertebral Manipulation. Butterworth, London, 1968.

chapter 6

Clinical application of spinal manipulation

This chapter will attempt to outline some guidelines which will help the operator to select the appropriate technique for each case. The approach to clinical application will be dichotomized into two major categories: the gentler techniques represented by the oscillatory techniques, and the more powerful techniques by the manipulative thrusts. An attempt will also be made to discuss how patients and symptoms react to manipulative treatment and the implications of this for the operator, how long and how often the patient should be treated, psychological handling of the treatment situation, recording of treatments and the dangers and contraindications of manipulation.

SELECTION OF TECHNIQUES

The question that often confronts the novice after examining a patient is "What do I do now?". An important prerequisite before the application of manipulation can yield the desired result is a logical, analytical and alert mind. There are some practitioners who have a stock of two of three techniques for each region of the spine and they apply these techniques in a set order regardless of the signs and symptoms which the patient has. And then they wonder why they are not getting results! How could they? Eventually, they turn around and blame the treatment instead of themselves. Selection of a particular technique is a result of a correct assessment of the patient's signs and symptoms followed by an evolution of the appropriate plan of treatment for that particular case. A change of technique from one to another is determined by the reaction of the signs and symptoms to previous treatment. This rule must be followed for the achievement of success and for the sake of safety. When the operator uses a particular technique with no change in the patient's condition, the technique should be performed again more firmly, and if the status quo still remains, it should be discarded for another technique. Repetition of a chosen technique should follow an improvement resulting from the use of it. If the chosen technique has exacerbated the patient's symptoms it should be discarded. It may of course be used in the future if the signs and symptoms demand it at that time.

It can be seen, therefore, that the application of manipulative treatment is hardly a hit-or-miss affair as it is regarded in some quarters. On the contrary, it is a product of logical reasoning and careful thinking. Personal experience is also an important feature. Some operators swear by some techniques while others do not care for them. This is why certain guidelines should be put in a broad perspective and laced with a degree of malleability.

The clinical application of manipulative treatment can be likened to a chess game. The opponents are the operator and the patient's symptoms. As the symptoms make their move the operator has to make a countermove not only to nullify the move of the former but also to establish a vantage position. Each case, therefore, in the treatment situation demands a particular maneuver and its own peculiar needs must be met with the appropriate approach.

One has to keep in mind that sometimes the right choice of technique may be made, but as a result of the operator's lack of expertise with regard to execution, the wrong amplitude of movement may be used or the joint may be moved in the wrong direction. Either of these factors will lead to a negative result or even to a worsening of the patient's condition.

Success in the use of manipulation is, therefore, a complex, multi-factorial affair.

APPLICATION OF OSCILLATORY TECHNIQUES

Many people associate the effectiveness of a manipulative technique with the flamboyance or force with which it is administered. This is a fallacy. Most patients who exhibit indications for manipulation require only the simpler, undramatic manipulative techniques in the form of oscillatory techniques. From the author's experience, 75 per cent of patients who are candidates for manipulative therapy can be helped with oscillatory techniques. It is only the remaining 25 per cent who need manipulative thrusts (see Figures 6.1 and 6.2).

Therefore, it stands to reason that the neophyte manipulator needs to acquire proficiency in the use of the gentler oscillatory techniques before he tries to learn the more difficult manipulative thrusts. From the point of view of learning progression, proficiency in the use of manipulative thrusts would depend on proficiency in the use of the oscillatory techniques.

Probably the most important factor in acquiring skill with oscillatory

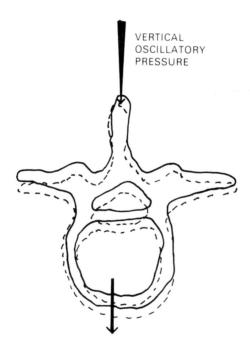

VERTICAL
OSCILLATORY
PRESSURE

FIG. 6.1. Effect of vertical oscillatory pressure. Broken lines show the position assumed by the vertebra after the application of pressure. Note the vertical movement of the vertebra.

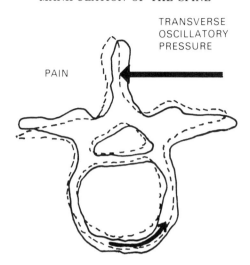

TRANSVERSE
OSCILLATORY
PRESSURE

PAIN

FIG. 6.2. Effect of transverse oscillatory pressure. Broken lines show the position assumed by the vertebra after the application of pressure. Note that the body of the vertebra tends to rotate away from the side of pain when pressure is applied on the spinous process toward the side of pain.

techniques is the ability to feel joint movement accurately. It is almost an art. It is something that comes with personal aptitude, practice and probably some natural talent. One can liken it to the delicate manner with which a professional safecracker manipulates a safe lock. It is unfortunate though that his talent is misdirected!

Oscillatory movement comprises a back and forth movement of low amplitude administered for about 15 to 30 seconds each time for two or three times depending on the acuteness of the symptoms, the reaction of symptoms and tolerance of the patient. The oscillation is effected by leading the joint to the point where pain is elicited and then leading it back to the starting point. An attempt should be made to achieve a state of resonance with the natural oscillatory frequency of the part under treatment. When using especially strong oscillatory rotatory techniques the natural oscillatory frequency tends to be fast for patients with ecto-morphic characteristics and slow for those with endomorphic features. The greater the amplitude of movement, the slower will be the rate of oscillation. It is the converse for smaller amplitudes. The integration of a smooth flow of movement, amplitude, velocity and rhythm is the impor-tant ingredient for a good and effective oscillatory technique.

When the pressure-release sequence has to be used, the thumbs consti-tute an intermediary between the operator's trunk and arms. The use of the intrinsics of the hand will lead to a poor technique because these muscles tire quickly, the operator's hands develop tension, rhythm is

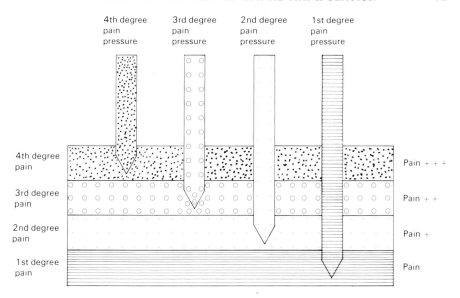

4th degree pain pressure   3rd degree pain pressure   2nd degree pain pressure   1st degree pain pressure

4th degree pain

3rd degree pain

2nd degree pain

1st degree pain

Pain + + +

Pain + +

Pain +

Pain

FIG. 6.3. Application of oscillatory techniques. The figure illustrates the concept of applying the right degree of pressure to the condition under consideration. The joint is led to the point where pain is elicited and not beyond it. The figure shows an arbitrary division of the joint range into four strata which represent degrees of pain. (Fourth-degree pain is high intensity and first-degree pain is low intensity.) Arrows represent pressure. Note that the operator has to lead the joint further in the use of first-degree pain and only a relatively little distance when dealing with fourth-degree pain. This concept also applies to the execution of oscillatory rotation.

lost, and the patient becomes uncomfortable. The overall result is an ineffective treatment.

The determinant of the depth of an oscillatory movement is pain and/or spasm. When the patient's pain is not too pronounced the operator can usually move the joint much farther before pain is elicited. When the pain is acute and the joint is very "touchy" the operator only has to move the joint a little distance before the patient reports pain. The right depth therefore has to be used for each case. Figure 6.3 illustrates this point.

As the operator nudges into the patient's pain during oscillatory movements the pain reacts in one of three ways.

1. The patient may report the easing of his pain. This is an encouraging sign. At this point the operator should increase the depth of the oscillatory movement as if he were "chasing" after the pain. This type of response on the part of the operator is maintained until the pain intensity remains static.

2. Not infrequently, the patient may report that there is no change one

way or the other in his pain even after about 20 to 25 seconds of continuous oscillations. In this case the same depth of movement is maintained.

3. The patient may complain that his pain is being exacerbated or sometimes he may add that there is pain shooting down to the dermatome of the vertebral level under manipulation. In this case the operator should reduce the depth of the movements. However, if the exacerbation continues the oscillatory movements should be discarded for another.

The various directions of oscillatory movements can always be changed if one does not obtain the desired result. The only exception is rotation of the head and neck, which should always be performed away from the side of pain. Diagrams 1–3 summarize the types of oscillatory techniques to be used in order of preference for bilaterally and unilaterally distributed symptoms with the directions of movement for the cervical, thoracic and lumbar regions. The order of preference, which goes from Diagram 1 to Diagram 3, has been arrived at after an analysis of the records of patients treated by the author. It should be regarded as a guide only.

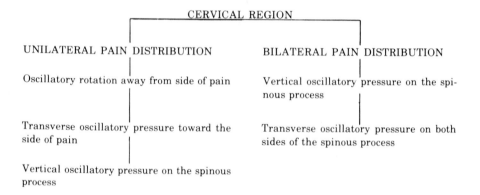

DIAGRAM 1

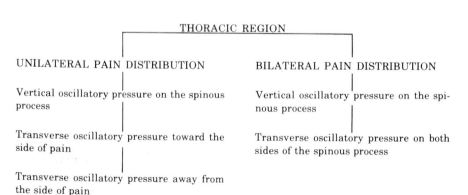

DIAGRAM 2

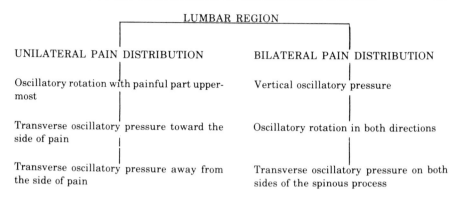

DIAGRAM 3

APPLICATION OF MANIPULATIVE THRUSTS

Earlier, it was pointed out that most patients usually respond to the gentler oscillatory techniques. When does one use the more powerful manipulative thrusts? There are two situations when they are warranted. Firstly, after the progressive improvement of a patient following oscillatory techniques a stalemate sometimes results between the operator and the patient's symptoms. Manipulative thrust then becomes indicated to clear the offending joint and to alter the status quo. Secondly, manipulative thrust is indicated when the patient's pain is minimal. Manipulative thrust is certainly not indicated when the patient has acute pain. Restoration of the general mobility of a joint can usually be effected by the application of the manipulative thrust in one plane.

The actual thrust is preceded by taking up all slack present in the joint. The manipulation is a high velocity movement but the operator should not lose sight of the fact that the movement is also of low amplitude. The direction of movement is opposite to the painful movement. This is consistent with Maigne's "concept of painlessness and opposite motion." [1-4] The direction, amplitude and velocity of the thrust should be accompanied by precision. The manipulative force should be focused on the joint to be manipulated when using specific techniques, while at the same time protecting the neighboring joints. As mentioned above, the operator should not commence the thrust until he can feel the necessary amount of tissue tension. This is very tricky. The tendency to administer the manipulative thrust prematurely is very real. When that happens the operator merely forces a movement which is present, and nothing is achieved. The ability to sense the exact amount of tissue tension required and to apply the thrust at the psychological moment is what differentiates the artist from the novice.

The operator must try to imagine the joints lying under his fingers as if he had X-ray eyes! He should direct his thrust in a perpendicular manner or along the same plane as the joint surface. Force should be avoided. The minimal force consistent with the achievement of maximal effect should be utilized. The manipulative thrust should finally be administered when the operator has no doubt in his mind that the right choice of technique has been made.

VACUUM SNAPS

This is the term often used to describe the "cracking" and "clicking" sounds which often accompany manipulative thrusts. A wealth of theories have been advanced by many authors to explain their origins.

Mennell's explanation is that these sounds are a result of sudden stretching of the joint capsule.[5] This causes a vacuum to be created, resulting in the capsule being drawn inward, precipitating the characteristic crack-like sound.

Fisk mentions the breaking of the joint seal.[6] A suction force is required to cause a separation of the joint surfaces, and in the process, the fluid on the joint surface is vaporized with the cracking of a film of nitrogen, producing the noise which the operator hears during a manipulative thrust. A reabsorption of the nitrogen has to take place before the event can be repeated, such as in the time delay one experiences after cracking one's fingers before the event can be repeated.

Maigne has theorized that the noise is attributable to the stretch imparted on the joint, causing a reduction of pressure on the synovial fluid,[4] which encourages the formation of gas bubbles within the fluid. It is the bursting of these gas bubbles which makes the noise.

Wright's explanation is that there is a breaking down of adhesions between articular surfaces.[7]

In 1947 Roston and Haines obtained a cracking sound after applying 8 kilograms to the finger.[8] A radiographic study done immediately after the sound showed a space between the two bones concerned. Their interpretation of their findings was that a partial vacuum was being formed as a result of the bony separation.

In clinical practice the operator has to remember that this cracking or clicking sound does not necessarily mean that a therapeutic effect has been achieved even though many patients usually look forward to it. It is reassuring to them and satisfying to the operator's ears.

REACTION OF PATIENTS, SIGNS AND SYMPTOMS TO TREATMENT

Different patients and various signs and symptoms do not react to or tolerate manipulative therapy in the same ways. For example, people who have a heavy build, or endomorphs, tend to tolerate both the frequency and intensity of manipulative treatments better than subjects who are slightly built, or ectomorphs.

After sessions of manipulative treatment about half of the patients treated will report treatment pain which continues for a variable period. Invariably it settles down by the time the patient arrives for the next session if he is on an every-other-day schedule. For patients who are scheduled for daily treatment it is not unusual to see some who still have treatment pain when they are seen the following day. The more intense the original pain, the greater the tendency for treatment pain to last longer. As treatment progresses successfully both the frequency and duration of this post-manipulative pain diminish.

Some detractors of manipulation sometimes point to the fact that effects of manipulation are only ephemeral. There may be an iota of truth in the charge. Apart from the various factors which have been discussed earlier, one reason for the return or the persistence of symptoms after manipulation is that there may be areas of muscle spasm which are secondary by-products of the primary joint lesion. Palpation of these areas reveals tightness and what used to be called "fibrositic nodules." Areas manifesting these characteristics are often the upper parts of the scapulae and muscles in the proximity of the vertebral borders, but they could be anywhere in the back. These areas should be treated with deep effleurage and pettrisage. The pettrisage should involve lifting of the skin and underlying muscle, rolling, squeezing and kneading. These massage techniques can be preceded with some form of heat therapy.

The application of the correct technique is sometimes not a guarantee of a quick success. This is because in certain conditions the patient should be expected to make slow progress. The following are some situations wherein the operator and patient should expect results to be slow in forthcoming: (1) if the patient exhibits a sciatic scoliosis and the convexity of the curve is on the painful side; (2) when the natural cervical or lumbar lordosis has disappeared because of pain or spasm; (3) when the straight-leg-raising test shows that there is a severe limitation of movement; (4) when pain shoots down the limbs as the patient is asked to extend the spine; (5) when the patient has very severe pain; (6) if the patient is relatively young (teenagers or younger patients); (7) when the symptoms are emanating from L3/4 or S1/S2 joints.

CERVICAL HEADACHES

This section deals with the origin of cervical headaches and their treatment with manipulation. The cervical origin of headaches is often puzzling to many practitioners. One has to realize that the greater occipital nerve which supplies the back of the head is derived from the second cervical root. In addition, the spinal nucleus of the trigeminal nerve is represented by an ophthalmic branch which goes down to the same level in the spinal cord as the greater occipital nerve.[9] The head itself derives its neurological formation from the first and second cervical segments. It is not surprising, therefore, that a lesion existing in either the occipito-atlantal joint or atlanto-axial joint will cause pain in any part of the head.

Maigne has emphasized the cervical source of headaches.[10] He mentions that these cervical headaches are usually one-sided and supraorbital and sometimes occipital on the same side. He also mentions the susceptibility of these headaches to manipulative treatment even after they have proved resistant to other forms of therapy. Braaf and Rossner conducted a 14-year study of 2000 patients reporting chronic recurring headaches.[11] Previously these patients' conditions had been diagnosed as post-concussion syndromes, idiopathic headaches, sinus headaches and so on. Their findings showed that 90 per cent of these patients' problems had to do with irritation of the cervical roots which had been precipitated by trauma in the past. Brain has drawn attention to the fact that extracranial structures may constitute the source of headaches with particular reference to the joints of the upper parts of the neck and the sensory nerves in that area.[12]

Headaches of cervical origin respond very well to vertical oscillatory pressure on the appropriate vertebral level, whether the distribution of symptoms is unilateral or bilateral. This technique should be tried first, and only if it is not successful should the usual rules regarding the application of techniques as discussed be followed.

DURATION AND FREQUENCY OF TREATMENT

How much treatment should a patient get? This varies from patient to patient and there is no clear-cut answer. If the signs and symptoms which the patient brings into the treatment room are recent and not very acute, a few treatments or sometimes one treatment will do the trick. On the other hand, a chronic case or symptoms which are very acute may require a relatively long time to deal with. When the patient has very acute pain, daily treatment is in order. This may be reduced to every other day depending on rate of progress and the presence or absence of treatment pain resulting from tissue reaction from previous treatment. This pain should be allowed to wear off before another treatment is administered, or it will mask the true clinical picture, making it difficult to assess properly the actual status of the patient's symptoms. Therefore, the frequency with which a patient is treated will depend very much on the findings of the operator at any one time.

An oscillatory technique can be repeated the number of times the patient can take it, usually two to five times. A manipulative thrust, however, is performed only once in a session. On the average it takes about four sessions of manipulative therapy to achieve maximal effect. If a patient has had about eight, nine or 10 sessions of treatment and the operator feels that he is not getting anywhere, the patient should be laid off and reassessed in about a week's time. Whether to reinstate or discontinue the treatment will depend on many factors including the operator's discretion. Not infrequently a patient may show up after the lay-off period reporting that he had never felt better in his life. This is because improvements are sometimes "latent" and do not manifest themselves until after a while. When there are no more symptoms treatment should be suspended.

As a last point, it has to be mentioned that there is a ceiling which cannot be exceeded as far as improvement goes during a particular session. When the operator hits this ceiling, further treatment will be considered overenthusiastic and unwise, and will result in the nullification of improvement obtained and possibly exacerbation of symptoms. A very "touchy" joint should not be treated with more than two sets of oscillatory movements, each lasting not more than 30 seconds. With joints which are not very painful five sets of oscillatory movements should be the maximum, with each set not lasting more than 30 seconds.

RECORDING OF TREATMENTS

After the application of treatments, records of the techniques used, how many times applied, the effects obtained and the reaction of the patient himself should be made. These records can act as an on-the-spot reminder when the patient arrives for his next session. It also helps to maintain a systematic approach toward helping the patient—a technique which was recorded as successful in the previous session can be repeated in the present session.

To reduce the secretarial tedium, abbreviations can be used to describe the type of technique used and what effect it had. For instance, if the operator administered vertical oscillatory pressure to a C5/6 joint two times and this was followed by relief of pain and increase of cervical mobility in external rotation and extension to the right, it can be written thus:

VOP——C5/6——2ce: Pain relieved: Ext. & rot. (R) > before

This of course is a sample of the author's shorthand method. The reader can always invent a system he finds convenient.

THE OPERATOR/PATIENT RELATIONSHIP

During application of manipulative therapy it is of paramount importance that the patient is made to relax as much as possible. One reason for the patient finding it difficult to relax is his feeling of apprehension. He wonders what the operator is about to do, especially if it is his first visit. An easy manner, gentle handling of the patient, a cheerful face, an optimistic although realistic outlook and an air of confidence will go a long way in making the patient "trust" the operator. The operator/patient rapport must be complete. The operator should be sympathetic, empathetic, unhurried and a good listener. The patient's realization that the operator "cares" helps enormously to let the patient put himself in the hands of the operator.

When the operator actually lays his hands on the patient's back, these hands should be able to communicate the qualities mentioned above. The patient, who is the consumer in this instance, can easily differentiate a rough and prodding hand or one which is unsure from a hand which is gentle, precise and which zeroes in on the problem, all of which will make the patient decide whether or not the operator "knows what he is doing."

DANGERS AND CONTRAINDICATIONS OF MANIPULATION

A search of literature on manipulation will reveal an interminable list of contraindications and warnings about the dangers ever attendant on this form of therapy. The end result is a confusing picture. Many authors have given accounts of the untoward effects of manipulation.

Hooper has reported two cases of posterior sequestration of lumbar intervertebral discs giving rise to paraparesis after they were treated with manipulation.[13]

Livingston mentions the result of a team study which had to do with the records of frequency of trauma in connection with manipulative therapy over a 3-year period of general practice.[14] During this period 676 patients who presented symptoms of spinal origin were examined. Of this number, 172 had made visits to chiropractors at some time. Out of these, 12 patients showed evidence of having suffered injury.

Maigne points out that vertebro-basilar accidents comprise the most severe complications of manipulative therapy.[15] However, he also emphasizes their rarity, considering the number of manipulations performed every day by practitioners.

An account of two cases of neurological damage following cervical manipulation has been given by Smith and Estridge.[16] One of the patients who had chiropractic manipulation went into a state of coma during the second session and died 3 days later. The second patient who also had manipulation developed headache and lost his ability to walk. Although his neurological deficits were rectified after 4 years, his headache persisted.

Blaine describes a case of anterior subluxation of the atlas after chiropractic manipulation.[17]

Fisher has described a cauda equina syndrome which resulted from "chiropractic adjustment."[18]

Despite the fact that many authors have pointed out injuries resulting from manipulative therapy, lack of manipulation may sometimes constitute a danger.[19] After examining the records of 10,000 patients treated over a 15-year period, Maigne mentions that there was not one single undesirable result.[4] Kuhlendahl and Hansell state that damage has been done to patients on certain occasions but this has been due to the fact that the manipulations were performed under wrong conditions by relatively untrained operators or by a physician who manipulated the patient under general anesthesia.[20] Paris states that in his clinical experience only 5 out of 1000 patients had symptoms which were exacerbated permanently or temporarily by manipulative therapy.[21] These values are, by a strange coincidence, similar to the values from the author's records. Even though deaths have occurred following manipulations it has to be pointed out that the number of manipulations carried out daily when compared to the mortality rate is indeed negligible.[22] In addition, one has to remember that the types of manipulations referred to in the above literature refer to manipulative thrusts and similar techniques.

When examining the considerations which influence contraindications, one is confronted with problems of defining the situation. For example, there are many conditions which are defined as contraindications because manipulation might cause damage. In some cases it is because manipulation will not affect the condition under consideration. Another factor is that manipulation may be contraindicated because the operator is considering using the more powerful manipulative thrusts while this problem may become irrelevant if the operator is intending to use oscillatory techniques. An example is the case of a patient who has nerve root compression, causing reflex activity dysfunction or loss of muscle power. In this case a manipulative thrust may not be indicated since the symptoms may be amenable to a gentle oscillatory technique. Each case deserves individual attention and the right approach.

There are of course some conditions which are absolute contraindications for both oscillatory techniques and manipulative thrusts, such as malignancy, osteomyelitis, fracture, infection, fever, renal disease or a disease simulating back symptoms.

Some conditions may be called contraindications but they are subject to the patient's condition, pain intensity, extent of disease, and the operator's discretion. Examples are: Paget's disease, rheumatoid arthritis, ankylosing spondylitis, vertebral artery involvement, osteoporosis, cauda equina syndrome, Scheuermann's disease. Other such contraindications include: (1) disturbance of micturition, saddle anesthesia and other signs suggesting that the third and fourth sacral roots are being compromised. (2) Pregnancy. After 4 months of pregnancy, it is wise to use techniques which involve sitting, side-lying or in some cases supine-lying only. During the 9th month of pregnancy, manipulative therapy may become impracticable. (3) Post-spinal operations. Manipulations rarely succeed after recurrence of pain following a laminectomy. This does not prevent the operator from trying anyway. In cases of spinal fusion, even oscillatory techniques may not be indicated. (4) Vertebro-basilar insufficiency, giving rise to "drop attacks" when the patient rotates his neck. Rotation and extension of the neck will cause circulatory arrest in the vertebral artery lying in the opposite side. When an abnormal vascular condition is present which causes a diminution of blood supply to a cerebral area, the situation becomes worse. In this case it may be wise to use those oscillatory techniques which involve pressure and avoid the rotatory ones. If the patient reports dizziness or vertigo during treatment of the neck area the treatment should be stopped. (5) The hypermobile joint. When an intervertebral joint shows limitation of movement, the ligaments of the joints lying superiorly will show a tendency toward overstretching as time goes by. This is in compensation for the hypomobility below. When this area of the back is treated with non-specific manipulation there is often an insufficient force to move the hypomobile level and the manipulation only helps to stretch the hypermobile level further. (6) Cord signs with the patient complaining of pins and needles in all four limbs.

The following are some closing remarks regarding dangers and contraindications of manipulative therapy.

1. The magnitude of the dangers of manipulation exhibit a positive correlation to the magnitude of the strength of the technique used.

2. When cervical rotation is employed in the presence of rheumatoid arthritis, the danger of rupture of the transverse and alar ligaments is very real, so also is the precipitation of atlanto-axial dislocation. It has to be remembered that rheumatoid arthritis causes the laxity of the atlanto-axial ligament and the erosion of the odontoid peg.

3. An osteoporotic rib can be fractured when a powerful rib pressure is employed in the manipulation of a costo-vertebral joint.

4. When the cervical region is manipulated in the face of contraindications the sequelae in the form of headaches and dizziness, for instance, are usually very difficult to relieve.

PREREQUISITES FOR A SAFE AND SUCCESSFUL MANIPULATION

This chapter will close with a list of the various factors which have been mentioned earlier and which the operator must always bear in mind for safety and success to be guaranteed.

1. Develop a sensitivity for tissue tension and joint movement.
2. Relax the patient.
3. Localize a manipulative force to the intended joint.
4. Manipulate the patient only after evaluating his signs and symptoms.

5. Base the selection of techniques on signs and symptoms. Reassess the patient after the application of each technique so that the next step will be determined by the patient's response to a previous technique.

6. Start gently, feeling your way through. Use manipulative thrusts only when the gentle techniques have outlived their usefulness and when there is minimal pain with joint stiffness.

7. Remember contraindications.

8. If one technique is proving its worth continue to use it until it is no longer effective.

9. Do not repeat any technique which causes dizziness or similar effects.

10. After each technique, have the patient sit up and assess the effect.

11. Direction of manipulative thrusts should show accuracy and precision. If specific, they should either be at right angles to the joint surfaces or along the planes of the joint surfaces being manipulated.

12. The amplitude and velocity of manipulative thrusts must be such that maximal effect is achieved with minimal effort.

13. Do not apply a manipulative thrust except when you are sure that the right technique has been selected.

14. Never push through spasm.

15. When the patient is free of all signs and symptoms treatment should be stopped.

REFERENCES

1. Maigne, R. *Les Manipulations Vertebrales*. Expansion Scientifique Française, Paris, 1960.
2. Maigne, R. The concept of painlessness and opposite motion in spinal manipulations (Translanted from French). Am. J. Phys. Med., *44:* 55–69, 1965.
3. Maigne, R. Le choix des manipulations dans le traitement des scientifiques. Rev. Rheum., *32:* 366–372, 1965.
4. Maigne, R. *Orthopedic Medicine. A New Approach to Vertebral Manipulation*. (Liberson, W. T., Ed. and Trans.) Charles C Thomas, Springfield, Illinois, 1972.
5. Mennell, J. *Back Pain*. Little, Brown, Boston, 1961.
6. Fisk, J. W. Manipulation in general practice. N. Z. Med. J., *74:* 172–175, 1971.
7. Wright, J. Mechanics in relation to derangement of the facet joints of the spine. Arch. Phys. Ther., *25:* 201–206, 1944.
8. Roston, J. B. and Wheeler, H. R. Cracking in the metacarpo-phalangeal joint. J. Anat., *81:* 165, 1947.
9. Chusid, J. G. *Correlative Neuroanatomy and Functional Neurology*. Lange Medical Publications, Los Altos, California, 1970.
10. Maigne, R. La cephalae suborbitaire sa frequente origine cervicale son traitement par manipulations. Ann. Med. Phys., *11:* 241–246, 1968.
11. Braaf, M. M. and Rossner, S. Chronic headaches. A study of over 2,000 cases. N. Y. State J. Med., *60:* 3987–3994, 1960.
12. Brain, Sir Russell. The treatment of pain. S. Afr. Med. J., *31:* 973, 1957.
13. Hooper, J. Low back pain and manipulation. Paraparesis after treatment of low back pain by physical methods. Med. J. Aust., *1:* 549–551, 1973.
14. Livingston, M. Spinal manipulation causing injury. Br. Columbia Med. J., *14:* 78–81, 1972.
15. Maigne, R. Les manipulations vertebrales et les thromboses vertebro basilaires. Angeiologie, *21:* 287–288, 1969.
16. Smith, R. A. and Estridge, M. N. Neurological complications of head and neck manipulations. Report of two cases. J. A. M. A., *182:* 528–531, 1962.
17. Blaine, E. S. Manipulative (chiropractic) dislocation of the atlas. J. A. M. A., *85:* 1356–1358, 1925.
18. Fisher, E. D. Report of a case of ruptured intervertebral disc following chiropractic manipulation. Kentucky Med. J., *41:* 14–18, 1943.
19. Cyriax, J. *Textbook of Orthopaedic Medicine*, vol. 1. Cassell, London, 1962.
20. Kuhlendahl, H. and Hansell, V. Nil nocere. Shaden bei wirbelsäulenreposition in norkose. Munch. Med. Weschr., *100:* 1738, 1958.
21. Paris, S. V. *Spinal Lesion*. Pegasus Press, Christchurch, New Zealand, 1965.
22. Brewerton, D. A. Conservative treatment of painful neck. Proc. R. Soc. Med., *57:* 163, 1964.

chapter 7 Traction

Traction can be regarded as a form of manipulative therapy since it involves the passive movement of joints either by a manual or mechanical agent.

The use of traction in treating neck and back pain is a recent development. Prior to 1900, traction figured in attempts to treat fractures, deformities of the spine and in some cases of dislocations. The inclusion of traction into the armamentarium of physical modalities for treating pain of spinal origin has been due to a mechanistic orientation toward pain causation in the spine which took place in the 1930s and which persists until today.

The reader who is interested in the history of traction will be fascinated by the book *Chirurgia* by Guido Guidi.[1] It includes Niketas' translations of Hippocrates, Galen and Oreibasius from Greek to Latin. The author, a 16th-century Florentine, had the honor of being the first professor of medicine in the College of the Medical Schools of France in Paris. Figure 7.1 is a reproduction from *Chirurgia*.

Spinal traction can be described as a force applied longitudinally to the spine, usually to a part of it to cause vertebral distraction. For the traction to be effective the force applied must exceed the friction offered by the part being treated.[2] When traction is applied to a recumbent body

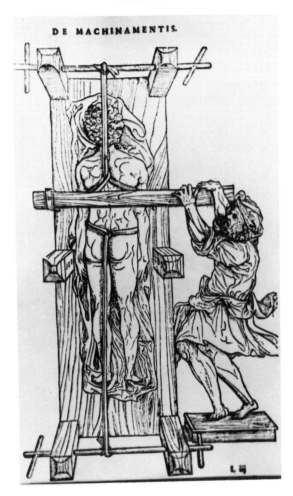

FIG. 7.1. Application of spinal traction for a gibbus. From Guido Guidi's *Chirurgia*, p. 529.

the applied force must exceed the friction of the part which lies between the applied force and the spinal area where the effect of the traction is desired.[3] The implication of this mechanical principle is clear. When traction is to be applied to the lumbar region, for instance, allowance must be made for the tractive force necessary to overcome the friction offered by the lower limbs and the pelvis.

Traction therapy can be administered to the spine by any of four methods.

1. Continuous application while the patient is on bed rest.

2. Sustained traction in which traction is applied for a specific duration of time, perhaps 10 minutes at a sitting.

3. Intermittent traction, entailing a gradual build-up of the tractive force to a certain poundage which is sustained for a while, followed by a gradual release until the poundage is reduced to zero. This process can be repeated a number of times during a session, the whole treatment lasting for about 10 to 15 minutes.

4. Rhythmic traction. This is almost identical to intermittent traction except that it is usually applied mechanically and sometimes with a rhythmic pattern developed for the particular patient under treatment.

Traction can be applied with the patient lying, sitting or standing. The positioning may also include some degree of flexion or extension of the spine. The sitting position during traction has the disadvantage of there being less stability of the trunk than during lying. But it offers less counter-resistance to the tractive force. When traction is applied in the sitting position and the tractive force is located under the chin, there is tendency for the head to be forced into extension. A pull located to the occiput, however, tends to force the head into flexion. This is also the tendency when traction is applied with the patient lying supine.

Cyriax has analyzed the effects of tractive force.[4] He mentions that traction induces a sub-atmospheric pressure during the longitudinal distraction of the vertebrae, which induces a centripetal effect. There is stretching of the posterior longitudinal ligament causing it to tighten and exert a centripetal force on a herniated disc.

Traction may be useful in clinical practice when manipulative techniques have not helped the patient. Some of the conditions which respond to traction are: osteoporosis, bilateral nerve root syndrome, symptoms resulting from S3/4 lesions and recent neurological changes of spinal origin. Judovich shows that for traction to be effective one had to apply 35 to 45 pounds for the cervical region, and 75 to 100 pounds for the lumbar region.[5, 6] Crisp discusses Christie's study of 60 patients who had back pain.[7] Fifty per cent of these patients were given traction therapy while the remaining 50 per cent were given placebo pills. Analysis of the results showed no difference in the treatments. Wilson advocates application of rotatory manipulation simultaneously with traction in the treatment of acute cervical disc syndrome.[8] Stoddard points out that rhythmic traction enhances the fluid exchange in the intervertebral discs.[9] It is, therefore, useful in treating conditions in which degenerative changes have taken place. Bourdillon examines the usefulness of traction in the management of acute back pain.[10] However, he does not share the belief that traction can reduce a herniated disc.

CERVICAL TRACTION

A cervical traction requires adjustability in two planes[11]—the length of the occipital and chin straps in the vertical direction and the distance between the occipital and chin straps in the horizontal direction. The various shapes of head and jaw need to be considered, including the relationship between the head and neck. Results of the study by De Sèze and Levernieux showed that a tractive force of 72 pounds achieved a distraction of 1.5 millimeters between each cervical vertebra and the next.[12] The application of 45 pounds by Judovich produced a distraction of 5 millimeters in the interspace.[5] Cyriax needed 300 pounds of traction before he could produce a distraction of 2.5 millimeters in each joint space.[4] Crue's results showed that the diameter of the vertebral foramen formed by the fifth and sixth cervical vertebrae could be altered by 1.5 millimeters when measured in the vertical direction as the neck was moved from 10 degrees of extension to 20 degrees of flexion.[13]

There are two tests which can be administered to determine whether cervical traction can be of help in relieving a patient's symptoms: the pressure-on-the-head test, and the traction test.

Pressure-on-the-Head Test

The operator places his hands on top of the patient's head and applies a vertical pressure. If this exacerbates the patient's symptoms, it is likely that traction will help. Not infrequently, when the pressure is applied with the head deviated to the painful side, pain may shoot down or parasthesia may be produced down the peripheral distribution of the nerve root which is bearing the brunt of the pressure.

Traction Test

(See Figure 7.2.) The patient is asked to lie supine with her head extending beyond the table. The operator, who is standing at the head end of the table, supports the patient's head with his left hand and places his right hand on her chin. He gradually pulls on her head, applying a longitudinal stretch on the neck which is lying mid-way between full flexion and full extension. The pull is held for about 1 minute. The patient is then asked if her pain was decreased—that is, her local and referred pain if present. If her pain is exacerbated, traction is not indicated. A mollification of symptoms is an indication that traction therapy may help the patient.

The following are some of the various ways in which traction can be applied to the cervical region.

HORIZONTAL TRACTION

(See Figure 7.3.) The patient is asked to lie supine on the traction table with pillows under his head and neck. A head halter is applied and strapped under the patient's chin and occiput. A strip of foam rubber may be applied for a cushioning effect between the mandible and the halter. The straps on the halter are fixed to a spreader bar. From the middle of the spreader bar a cord leaves to pass over a pulley. The distal end of the cord is attached to a weight or to an electronic machine which can be employed to produce the necessary tractive force (Figure 7.4). Ideally, the

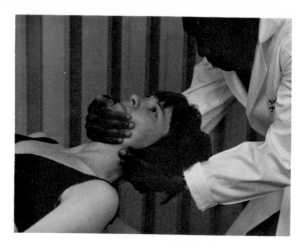

FIG. 7.2. Traction test with patient lying supine.

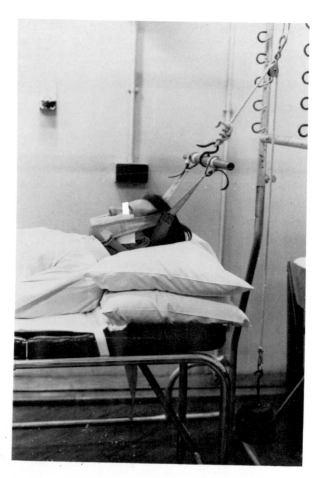

FIG. 7.3. Horizontal traction to the cervical region using pulley and weights.

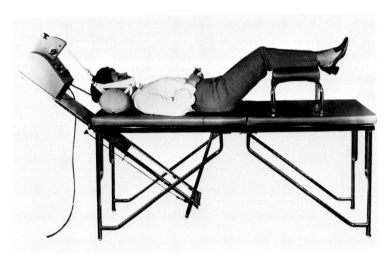

FIG. 7.4. Horizontal traction to the cervical region using an electronic device.
Courtesy of Tru-Eze Manufacturing Co., Inc., Burbank, California.

head and neck should make an angle of about 35 degrees with the plane of the body. This can be obtained by adjusting the thickness of pillow or pillows used. The poundage which can be used varies with each patient. The average weight is about 25 pounds. The duration of treatment also varies; an average would be 10 to 20 minutes. Weight and duration also depend on the patient's tolerance. The guiding principle should be to use the least poundage which affords maximal relief.

INTERMITTENT SUSTAINED CERVICAL TRACTION

(See Figure 7.5.) The patient is supine-lying with the head and neck on pillows. The head halter is applied and attached to a spreader bar between which there is a spring balance to record the amount of poundage being applied during traction. The operator pulls with the traction handle to the desired poundage, holds it for about 30 seconds and then gradually relaxes the pull. About 35 pounds would be ideal. The pull-relax sequence is repeated about five to seven times during a session. If symptoms are acute, daily treatment would be in order, reducing to every other day when the patient starts improving or if the symptoms were mild to begin with. Stoddard recommends this form of traction if the patient's symptoms are attributable to a congestive status of the intervertebral foramen and nerve root.[9] Because of movement which takes place during treatment, blood flow is enhanced and drainage improved.

CERVICAL TRACTION IN A SITTING POSITION

The patient is seated comfortably on a chair. The head halter is applied and attached to the spreader bar. The traction unit may be suspended

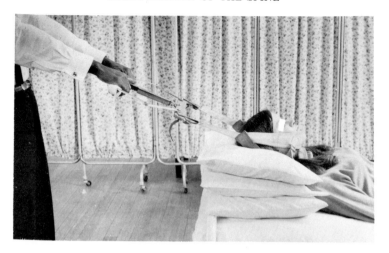

FIG. 7.5. Intermittent sustained cervical traction.

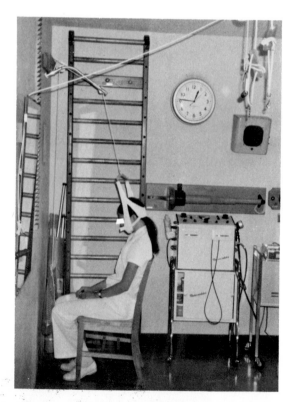

FIG. 7.6. Cervical traction in sitting position using an overhead traction unit.

from the top of a door or from a wooden fixture on the wall, as in Figure 7.6. The cord from the spreader bar is passed through a pulley system. The weight is hung from the standing length of the rope. Note that the weight used for the patient in Figure 7.6 is in the form of a graduated water bag positioned at the knee level. An electronic machine may be used to provide traction in the sitting position, as in Figure 7.7. The guidelines for poundage and duration of treatment are the same as for horizontal traction, however, relatively less poundage may be expected since the frictional force encountered in the case of horizontal traction would be more.

CERVICAL TRACTION IN A STANDING POSITION

(See Figure 7.8.) This is a method of traction seen by the author at the Fairview Hospital Physical Therapy Department, Minneapolis, Minne-

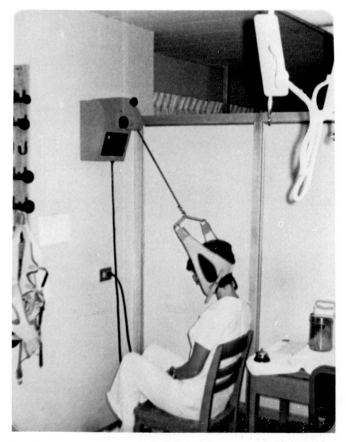

FIG. 7.7. Cervical traction in sitting position using an electronic machine.

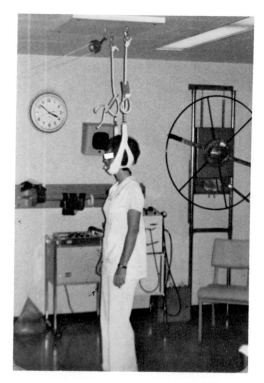

FIG. 7.8. Cervical traction in standing position.

sota. Two ropes are dropped from the ceiling where they are securely attached by hooks. The patient is asked to stand on a bathroom scale (Figure 7.9) between the cords which are attached to the head halter with which she has been fitted.

The patient uses her body weight to apply auto-traction. The operator takes note of the weight registered by the patient while she is standing on the scale. The patient is asked to bend her knees (Figure 7.10), and as she does, there is an upward pull from the head halter causing traction on the neck. Simultaneously, this relieves the weight which falls on the scale and it is registered accordingly. The difference between the pre-knee-bend and post-knee-bend weights registered is approximately the tractive force which falls on the neck.

As the patient moves forward, her head and neck will tend to move into extension and as she moves backward they will tend to move into flexion.

Poundage and duration will be dictated by the factors discussed earlier.

Certain categories of patients may find this form of traction therapy difficult to tolerate, including patients with painful knees, some elderly patients and patients who lack stability in standing due to a physical or neurological problem.

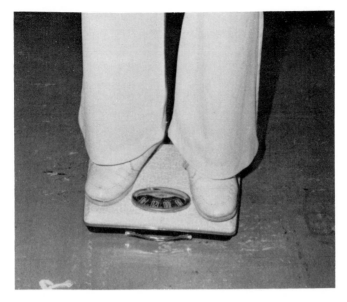

FIG. 7.9. Patient standing on a bathroom scale during application of cervical traction in standing position.

LUMBAR TRACTION

The application of lumbar traction requires basically a comfortable harness around the thorax and another around the pelvis (Figure 7.11). These two harnesses are attached to fixed points. The patient must also be made comfortable and relaxed. Some patients prefer having their hips and knees in flexed positions before they can relax (Figure 7.12). With the help of straps, the thoracic harness is attached to a fixed point behind the patient's head and the pelvic belt beyond the feet. Prior to the application of the tractive force all slack must be taken off the straps.

Most commercially marketed traction tables have static thoracic components with mobile lumbar components. Figure 7.11 shows a mobile thoracic component and a static lumbar component. Ideally the design of a lumbar traction table should be such that it affords movement of both components by rollers. Maitland has advocated the use of a friction-free traction table for two reasons.[14] One is that it is time-saving since the operator does not have to eliminate friction initially as with conventional tables. The other reason he states is that the small increases and decreases in the tractive force can be easily and accurately made with the comfortable knowledge that they are immediately effective in the lumbar spine.

Cords from lumbar harnesses are usually components of lumbar traction units. They pass over pulleys and screw threads to scales which measure the tractive force, or they may pass from the lumbar harness

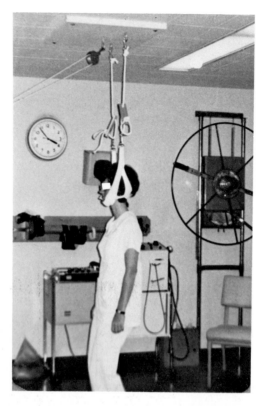

FIG. 7.10. Cervical traction in standing position. As patient bends at the knees there is an upward pull resulting in traction to the neck.

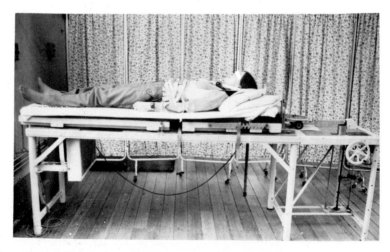

FIG. 7.11. Lumbar traction. Note the adjustable thoracic and pelvic harnesses which are attached to fixed points.

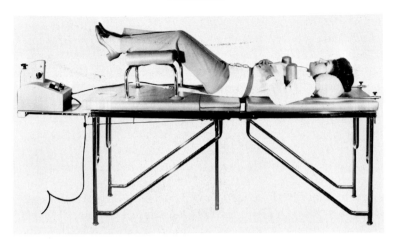

FIG. 7.12. Lumbar traction. Some patients prefer having their hips and knees in flexed positions before they can relax.
Courtesy of Tru-Eze Manufacturing Co., Inc., Burbank, California.

into an electronic machine which pulls according to what the operator has set (Figure 7.12).

If one position, for example, supine-lying, does not lead to improvement, prone-lying may be tried. If either position does not help, one may conclude that traction therapy is not the answer.

The pull applied should vary with each patient depending on the patient's tolerance. When the patient appears for treatment for the first time, a low poundage should be tried for a short duration. If the patient reports exacerbation of pain during the first session, the pull and duration should be reduced. The amount of pull should be maintained when improvement is reported. An average of 80 to 100 pounds for 10 to 20 minutes would be required. These values are rough estimates. The operator should remember that the scale should function merely as an indication of the amount which has been applied for record purposes. It is the patient's symptoms rather than the scale which dictate the amount of pull required. The operator should also keep in mind that the patient's post-traction therapy flexion is often temporarily more limited than what it was before treatment.

Taking down traction which has been set up should be done slowly. A sudden release of the traction may precipitate a sudden exacerbation of the patient's symptoms. A patient may also complain of vertigo or dizziness following traction, as a result of a shift in the cerebro-spinal fluid.

The rest of this chapter will review some of the literature on lumbar traction with regard to experimental works and conclusions which have emerged from them. A word will also be said about contraindications.

After his investigation of the physical principles of traction, Judovich concludes that 50 per cent of the weight of the body lay in the region of the third and fourth lumbar vertebrae.[6, 15] He referred to the practice of hanging 30-pound weights from the legs or pelvis as ineffective for producing traction to the lumbar region, because a pull which falls short of 25 per cent of the body weight is insufficient to have any effect in the lumbar region. He advocated the use of the split-table for the elimination of fraction.

Scott designed a traction frame which could be adjusted to alter the patient's position into more flexion or extension and to increase or decrease lateral deviation if traction were to be applied in side-lying.[16]

Masturzo, after the application of traction to the lumbar region through a pelvic and a thoracic corset, showed that the distance of the disc space increased by 1 millimeter in either direction.[17]

Hood and Chrisman investigated the effect of intermittent traction to the lumbar region in 40 patients[18] whose conditions had been diagnosed as herniation of intervertebral discs with sciatic symptoms in both legs and back pain. Of these patients, 21 showed good to excellent results according to the criteria which the investigators had established. Their conclusion was that lumbar traction was effective in the management of herniated intervertebral discs. The investigators also pointed out that traction had the effect of increasing the amount of space for the emerging nerve root through the intervertebral foramen.

Matthews investigated the effects of sustained traction with the help of epidurography.[19] He applied 120 pounds of traction to the lumbar region of his subjects. Among those who had sciatic symptoms but with no neurological deficits, the lumbar vertebrae showed evidence of distraction and the contrast which was used appeared sometimes to be sucked into the intervertebral disc space. The posterior aspects of the lumbar discs were outlined by the aid of epidural injections of contrast medium by Matthews and Yates.[20] X-rays of the lateral aspect of the spine were taken before, during and after the administration of traction to study its effects. The X-ray of one patient who did not have a disc prolapse showed no significant effect with traction. Two patients who had multiple disc protrusions showed evidence of the reduction of these by traction.

Weber gave 20 minutes of intermittent lumbar traction daily for 5 to 7 days to patients with sciatica and neurological signs.[21] The results of his study showed that there was no benefit with traction therapy.

CONTRAINDICATIONS OF TRACTION

Without cataloguing conditions which contraindicate traction, it would be sufficient to say that traction should not be applied in those conditions which contraindicate manipulative therapy. Apart from disease conditions which are an absolute bar, there are some situations in which traction cannot be given, such as cases in which patients exhibit signs of respiratory problems, development of claustrophobia under traction or an inability to tolerate traction because of nervousness. Patients who have developed extensive scarring in the abdominal region following surgery find it difficult to tolerate lumbar traction. When a patient demonstates hypomobility in the area of the spine under treatment, traction may prove ineffectual. In some cases some harm may even result, because the tractive force will act mainly on the hypermobile joint, which is usually a concomittant of hypomobility, causing a further strain on it without affecting the hypomobile segment.

REFERENCES

1. Guidi, G. *Chirurgia*. Paris, 1544.
2. Judovich, B. D. and Nobel, G. R. Traction therapy. A study of resistance forces. Am. J. Surg., *93:* 108, 1957.
3. Licht, S., Ed. *Massage, Manipulation and Traction*. Elizabeth Licht, New Haven, Connecticut, 1960.
4. Cyriax, J. *Textbook of Orthopaedic Medicine*, vol. I. Cassell, London, 1962.
5. Judovich, B. D. Herniated cervical disc—A new form of traction therapy. Am. J. Surg., *84:* 646, 1952.
6. Judovich, B. D. Lumbar traction therapy. A study of resistance forces. Lancet, *74:* 411, 1954.
7. Crisp, E. J. Discussion of the treatment of backache by traction. R. Soc. Med., *43:* 805, 1955.
8. Wilson, J. N. A simple traction harness for cervical manipulation. J. Bone Joint Surg., *39B:* 756–757, 1957.
9. Stoddard, A. *Manual of Osteopathic Technique*. Hutchinson, London, 1969.
10. Bourdillon, J. *Spinal Manipulation*. Heinemann, London, 1970.
11. Maitland, G. A cervical halter. Physiotherapy, *15:* 24, 1969.
12. De Sèze, M. and Levernieux, J. Précisions sur l'emploi des tractions vertébrales. Rev. Rheu., *17:* 303, 1950.
13. Crue, B. J. Importance of flexion in cervical traction for radiculitis. U.S.A.F. Med. J. *8:* 374, 1957.
14. Maitland, G. *Vertebral Manipulation*. Butterworth, London, 1964.
15. Judovich, B. D. Lumbar traction therapy—Elimination of physical factors that prevent lumbar stretch J. A. M. A., *159:* 549–550, 1955.
16. Scott, B. O. A universal traction frame and lumbar harness. Ann. Phys. Med., *2:* 258–260, 1955.
17. Masturzo, A. A vertebral traction for sciatica. Rheumatism, *11:* 62, 1955.
18. Hood, L. B. and Chrisman, D. Intermittent pelvic traction in the treatment of the ruptured intervertebral disk. J. Am. Phys. Ther. Assoc., *48:* 21–30, 1968.
19. Matthews, J. A. Dynamic discography: A study of lumbar traction. Ann. Phys. Med., *9:* 275–279, 1968.
20. Matthews, J. A. and Yates, D. A. Letter. Treatment of sciatica. Lancet, *1:* 352, 1974.
21. Weber, H. Traction therapy in sciatica due to disc prolapse. (Does traction treatment have any positive effect on patients suffering from sciatica caused by disc prolapse?) J. Oslo City Hosp., *23:* 167–176, 1973.

chapter 8

Case histories

The case histories which will be discussed in this chapter have been selected from the records of patients treated by the author. They will illustrate many of the points which have been mentioned in earlier chapters with regard to examination, execution of oscillatory techniques and manipulative thrusts. It is hoped that the discussion of these case histories will be of help to the experienced, neophyte and prospective manipulative therapists in the treatment situation. Only the salient points of the cases will be outlined. The procedures which will be discussed need not be followed rigidly when similar conditions for which they have been used are encountered. They are meant to act as guides. On the other hand one should bear in mind that there are certain basic principles which determine the selection and subsequent execution of most of the manipulative techniques.

CASE 1. CERVICAL HEADACHE

A 40-year-old housewife had been having a left-sided hemi-cranial headache for 6 years. The original diagnosis of her family doctor was "migraine." When the patient had acute attacks she suffered from blurred vision and nausea and on many occasions she was confined to bed until the attack subsided. Her doctor referred her to a neurologist, who, after conducting numerous tests, could not find a pathological basis for her problems. Because of his inability to establish the cause of these headaches, he sent the patient for manipulative therapy as an empirical measure.

Examination revealed severe tenderness over C1, C2 and C3 levels. The patient found rotation of her head and neck to the left almost impossible due to pain. Side flexion to the right side showed moderate limitation with some pain.

Vertical oscillatory pressure was administered to the tender vertebral levels during the first three sessions. This led to the improvement of side-flexion to the left and rotation to the left. The pain was also much reduced. On the fourth session the patient reported that the pain was greatly reduced in intensity and frequency, although she still had occasional headaches. Vertical oscillatory pressure was repeated, this time with increased vigor. On the fifth session the patient reported that she had had only a single brief attack since the last treatment session and that it had been mild. Her blurred vision and nausea had ceased. All neck movements had full range with the exception of rotation to the left which produced slight pain. A cervical rotatory thrust, first directed to the C1/C2 joint and then to the C2/C3 joint, was administered. When the patient arrived for treatment for the sixth session, not only had she not had any attack since the last treatment, but also all movements were full and pain-free. Treatment was discontinued.

The patient reappeared a month later complaining of recurring headaches, this time, in a mild form. Rotatory thrust to the right as performed before was again administered. The symptoms disappeared. The author corresponded with this patient 2 years later and all was well with her.

CASE 2. SEVERE NECK PAIN OF SUDDEN ONSET

A 35-year-old bank manager suddenly felt a "click" in this neck as he turned his head to look behind him while attempting to back up his car. The resulting pain was so agonizing that he had to stop his car for a while until it passed.

When he was seen in the examination room, his head and neck demonstrated a rotation deformity to the left. An attempt to perform voluntary rotation to the right proved futile because of pain. Pain was mainly located on the left side of his neck. The skin-roll test proved positive over C3, C4 and C5 levels.

On the patient's first visit his neck was treated with oscillatory rotation to the right for 20 seconds. On post-treatment assessment, the subjective and objective results were indifferent. The oscillatory rotation was repeated but there was no change. Because of the severity of the pain the patient was fitted with a cervical collar before he went home. During the second session the patient reported essentially no change in his pain. Transverse oscillatory pressure was administered to C3, C4 and C5 levels for 20 seconds each. The direction of the pressure was toward the left side. After treatment the neck showed 10-degree improvement in rotation to the right. This treatment was repeated. On the third visit, the patient reported that his neck was pain-free. On assessment of neck movements, there was no restriction in any direction except rotation to the right, which was short by about 5 degrees. He was removed from his cervical collar and treatment was discontinued under the assumption that the slight residual loss of movement would be restored with time.

CASE 3. DULL ACHE AT THE BACK OF THE NECK

A 50-year-old man had a history of pain at the back of his neck for 4 years. When it began, he thought that it was "fibrositis" and he often asked his wife to rub his neck with one of the popular ointments. Relief was often incomplete and ephemeral. Since its onset, the pain came and went in waves. It was particularly troublesome at nights, robbing the patient of sleep.

During examination the patient described the pain as dull and nagging in nature. All neck movements were equally limited and painful. Palpation revealed tenderness over the C3, C4, C5, C6 and C7 levels. The radiologist's report indicated degenerative changes at the C4/C5, C6/C7 and C7/C8 joints. Pain was usually of high intensity in the mornings, wearing off during the day, and building up again in the night.

The tender vertebral levels were treated with vertical oscillatory pressure. On assessment the patient reported that the neck felt "looser." Neck movements showed an increase in mobility. During the second session, vertical oscillatory pressure was repeated. After treatment all movements apart from flexion were short by only 15 degrees. Flexion was short by 20 degrees. During the third and fourth sessions vertical oscillatory pressure was again administered, with no objective or subjective change in signs and symptoms. During the fifth session the patient reported that apart from some soreness he had no pain. All neck movements now showed full mobility except for a 15-degree restriction in flexion. The patient was given microwave diathermy to the area of soreness. He was told to report back if the original symptoms returned. The author has not heard from him since then.

CASE 4. PAIN IN THE NECK WITH PAIN AND PARESTHESIA IN BOTH ARMS

A 45-year-old headmaster reported pain in this neck radiating down both arms. The pain in his neck had started about 4 years prior to examination as a dull ache. About 6 months prior to his examination he noticed pain shooting down his arms intermittently beginning with his right arm and then the left. Pain was often accompanied by odd sensations; sometimes there was numbness over his right thumb.

When he was examined, all of the patient's neck movements were painful in all directions. Neck extension caused pain to shoot down both arms. The triceps jerk on the right arm was diminished. Sensation was also diminished when the right thumb was pricked with a pin. The radiologist's report indicated gross degenerative changes at C4/C5, C5/C6 and C6/C7 joints. He was wearing a collar which his doctor had given him.

During the first visit, vertical oscillatory pressure was administered over C4, C5, C6 and C7. Each level was treated for 25 seconds. During the oscillations the patient reported pain shooting down his arms with every pressure, however, the intensity seemed to diminish as the treatment progressed. After treatment there was about a 10-degree gain in mobility in all neck movements. When the patient arrived for the second session he reported a diminution of pain both in his neck and arms. The gain in neck mobility from the previous session was still being maintained. Vertical oscillatory pressure was repeated. On the third visit there was no longer any pain in his left arm, and the pain in his right arm was much less. Vertical oscillatory pressure was again repeated. On the fourth visit there was slight pain in the right side of his neck and the right deltoid area. The numbness in his right thumb still seemed to be present. Oscillatory rotation to the left was administered for 25 seconds, and was repeated two times. This removed the pain from the right deltoid area. On the fifth session the patient reported that he felt much better. He had no pain in his arms. The residual pain which he had had in the right side of his neck was treated with a rotatory thrust first directed at the C3/C4 joint and then the C5/C6 joint. When the patient arrived for the sixth session he was completely pain-free. The numbness in the right thumb still persisted. Treatment was discontinued and the patient was asked to report back if he had a relapse. Nothing has been heard from him since.

CASE 5. "WHIPLASH" INJURY TO THE NECK

The car in which a 25-year-old housewife was driving was hit from behind by a heavy truck as she approached a traffic light. She remembered passing out for a while after the accident, followed by an excruciating pain in her neck. She was taken to the nearest hospital where she received emergency treatment and was given a cervical collar. She was referred 6 weeks later by her doctor for treatment.

When the patient was seen her whole neck was a mass of spasm after removal of the collar. Her neck was like a rigid pillar. Palpation over C2, C3, C4, C5 and C6 revealed extreme tenderness. The patient found it impossible to move her neck in any direction. The pain was diffuse but was particularly acute at the back of the neck.

During the first session the patient was given infra-red rays for 20 minutes for a sedative effect. However, her pain was so acute that she could not stand even the gentlest oscillatory maneuver. She was then treated with sustained-intermittent cervical traction. Five pulls were given, each sustained for 30 seconds with a maximal poundage of 35. After treatment the result was indifferent. During the second visit traction therapy was repeated, preceded by heat therapy as before. There was no appreciable difference in symptoms. During the third session the patient reported some improvement in her pain. After the administration of sustained-intermittent traction, vertical oscillatory pressure was applied to C2, C3, C4, C5 and C6. This was performed once on each level for a duration of 10 seconds each. On post-treatment assessment, apart from slight decrease in spasm there was essentially no change in symptoms. When the patient reported for treatment for the fourth session, she said that she had developed nausea and later vomited after the previous visit. Her pain had also worsened after leaving the clinic but it later decreased and was now showing improvement. On examination the spasm in her neck was markedly reduced. The heat treatment was repeated followed by sustained-intermittent cervical traction and vertical oscillatory pressure for 15 seconds on each level. This routine was repeated during the fifth and sixth sessions. When the patient arrived for the seventh session, all neck movements were nearly full except for a dull ache in the back of the neck. Vertical oscillatory pressure was applied to C3, C4, and C5 for 20 seconds each. This was repeated during the eighth and ninth sessions. On the 10th visit the patient reported a marked improvement in her pain. Spasm in her neck was minimal. Pain was also minimal. All movements were full except flexion and extension which were short by 10 degrees each.

Treatment was suspended for a period of 2 weeks. The patient was removed from her collar and asked to report back after the rest period. Meanwhile, her case was reviewed with her doctor as to discontinuation or reinstatement of therapy.

The patient telephoned the author 10 days later to say that her family was moving out of town because her husband was going into a new job. She wrote 2 months later to say that she still maintained the improvement resulting from the sessions of treatment, but had intermittent periods of dull ache at the back of her neck but that it was nothing to make a fuss about.

CASE 6. PAIN OF "STABBING" NATURE IN THE RIGHT SCAPULAR REGION

A woman of 40 felt a sharp pain in the right scapular region as she shouted at her husband during a family quarrel 2 weeks prior to her initial examination. After the incident she observed that the pain had increased in intensity and had spread to her right lower neck.

On examination, flexion, extension and side-flexion of her neck to the left and rotation to the right were all limited. These movements elicited a stabbing pain in the right scapular region. The patient said that the pain felt as if someone were digging a knife into her back. Palpation revealed tenderness over C6, C7, T1 and T2. The pain was usually ameliorated by activities which involved the upper limbs.

Oscillatory rotation was applied to the patient's neck for 20 seconds, repeated three times toward the left side. The oscillations were directed to the lower cervical region, followed by vertical oscillatory pressure applied to T1 and T2 for 20 seconds each, repeated two times. On post-treatment assessment, extension and side-flexion to the left improved and were now both limited by 10 degrees. On the second visit the stabbing pain had been replaced by a dull ache. Treatment as in the first visit was repeated. This restored full neck movements, however, side-flexion to the left and rotation to the right caused pain at the extremes of their ranges. Vertical oscillatory pressure was performed on T1 and T2 for 30 seconds each after which the pain disappeared at the extremes of rotation to the right and side-flexion to the left. The dull ache in the scapular region was still there. On the third visit the patient said she felt much relieved but wished she could get rid of the dull ache. The improvement in neck movements was still being maintained. Vertical oscillatory pressure as done in the prior visit was repeated with no appreciable difference in the ache. Transverse oscillatory pressure was applied to T1 and T2 levels. The direction was toward the right side. This was done for 25 seconds on each level, repeated two times. After this treatment, the pain disappeared. On the fourth visit the patient reported only residual aching in the same area. Transverse oscillatory pressure was repeated as for the last visit. The aching disappeared and the treatment session was concluded.

CASE 7. PAIN ACROSS THE BACK

A brick fell on the back of a 39-year-old mason at work. This was 1 year prior to his initial examination. Following the accident, he was treated in a hospital and the doctor ordered 7 days of rest from work. The radiograph showed no evidence of a fracture. The patient resumed work after the 7-day rest period, fully recovered from the pain resulting from the accident. However, about 2 weeks prior to his examination he started to experience what he described as "shooting" pain across his back. He said that it sometimes felt like a combination of an electric shock and pain darting transversely across the middle of his back.

Examination revealed tenderness and spasm over T4, T5, T6 and T7 levels. Rotation of the thoracic spine to the left and right was equally limited by about 30 degrees. Intervertebral joint mobility showed limitation at T4/T5 and T5/T6 joints during rotation to both sides.

During the first session treatment consisted of vertical oscillatory pressure performed on T4, T5, T6 and T7. During the oscillations the shooting pain was initially exacerbated followed by an abatement. The treatment was applied for 15 seconds on each level and repeated two times. On post-treatment assessment, rotation of the thoracic spine to the right and left increased by 20 degrees each but the patient complained of treatment pain. During the second visit, the patient reported that when he got home after the last treatment, he experienced an acute pain in his back. He said that it felt as if someone was driving a nail through his back. This subsided and was replaced by a feeling of relief which he still had at the time of the visit. The pain was still there but it was greatly reduced in intensity. Vertical oscillatory pressure was performed as before. On the third visit there was only a dull ache in the T6 region. Vertical oscillatory pressure was performed on T6 for 20 seconds, and repeated three times. When the patient appeared for the fourth session, he reported that virtually all of the pain in his back was gone except a slight ache which he felt at intervals in the T6 area. Vertical thrust was delivered on the T6/T7 joint once during which a clicking sound was heard, and on post-treatment assessment, the pain had disappeared. During the fourth visit the patient was completely pain-free. All movements were full and caused no pain. A short while before the visit he had seen his doctor who had given him permission to return to work. (A few days of rest from work before this time had been ordered.)

The patient telephoned for an appointment a month later because of relapse of pain. Vertical thrust was performed once and was followed by complete relief. After this session the patient was never heard from again.

CASE 8. PAIN IN THE LEFT SHOULDER AND LEFT SIDE OF THE CHEST

A 48-year-old draftsman developed pain in his left shoulder and in the left side of his chest about 2 years prior to his initial examination. Before the onset of these symptoms he had had slight pain and stiffness in his neck. The main source of worry for this patient was the chest pain, which he thought portended heart trouble. His family doctor, who had recorded negative findings in this direction, sent him to a cardiologist who, after running a few tests, also declared that the source of his problems was not his heart. Radiological studies of his left shoulder revealed nothing significant, but did indicate narrowing of C5/C6, C6/C7, T3/T4 and T5/T6 joints.

On examination, all neck movements were limited. Side-flexion to the left elicited pain in the left shoulder area, as did rotation to the left. Full neck extension was limited by 80 per cent and flexion and side-flexion to the left lacked 50 per cent of their ranges. The skin-roll test was positive over C5, C6, T3, T4 and T5 levels. Testing of intervertebral mobility revealed rotatory restriction to the left and right in T3/T4 and T4/T5 joints. The patient described the pain in the chest as "burning" and said it was particularly bad at night. The pain in his left shoulder was a constant dull ache of consistent intensity.

During the first session, oscillatory rotation was administered to the cervical area twice for a duration of 25 seconds each time. The direction of the rotation was toward the right side and the oscillations were directed to the lower cervical region. Vertical oscillatory pressure was applied to T3, T4, T5 and T6 levels for 20 seconds on each level, and was repeated two times. Following this treatment, pain in the shoulder seemed to diminish in intensity. Cervical rotation to both sides was almost full but there was no change in neck extension. During the second session the patient reported that his pain had decreased considerably. Treatment was repeated as for the first session but there was no change in symptoms. On the third visit the patient reported that he was completely pain-free. All movements were full except extension which was still limited by about 20 per cent and caused pain at the extreme. Vertical oscillatory pressure was applied to C5 and C6 for a duration of 30 seconds on each level and repeated three times. When the patient arrived for the fourth session, he was still pain-free but lacked 10 per cent of neck extension. Vertical oscillatory pressure was applied as for the prior visit, followed by restoration of full extension. By this time, the patient was symptom-free and treatment was discontinued.

CASE 9. "GIRDLE" PAIN AROUND THE TRUNK

Two months prior to her examination a 35-year-old housewife fell down at home, hitting her back against a piece of furniture. Apart from a slight discomfort in her back at the time of the accident, there was no serious pain and she soon forgot about the incident. Four days prior to examination, however, when she woke up in the morning, she felt a "gripping" pain which seemed to encircle her trunk. This pain seemed more pronounced on her right side than on her left, and was exacerbated by deep breathing and coughing.

When the patient was examined, there was tenderness over T6, T7 and T8. Rotation of the thoracic spine to the right side caused pain and was limited by 50 per cent. Rotation to the left was limited by 30 per cent. Side-flexion to the right and left was limited by 50 per cent in each direction. Forward flexion and extension were full and pain-free.

On the first session vertical oscillatory pressure was performed on T6, T7 and T8. The duration of treatment on each level was 25 seconds and was repeated three times. After treatment, full rotation to the left was restored and rotation to the right became limited by 30 per cent. When the patient was seen during the second session she reported that relief from pain after the last treatment lasted for about 5 hours after which it became so intense that she felt as if her trunk was being "gripped in a vise." This experience lasted for about 1 hour and then passed. At the time of the visit, the pain was much less intense and was mainly located on the right side. Vertical oscillatory pressure was administered as for the last visit. On post-treatment assessment, the pain on the right side assumed the nature of a dull ache. Side-flexion to the right and left was still short by 50 per cent each way. On the third visit the patient had maintained the improvement resulting from the last treatments. Her main problems now were limitation of side-flexion and pain on her right side. Vertical oscillatory pressure was administered as before but there was no change in her condition. Transverse oscillatory pressure was then performed on T6, T7 and T8. The direction of pressure was toward the right, repeated two times on each level, each time for a duration of 20 seconds. After treatment the dull ache on her right side was now hardly noticeable by the patient. Side-flexion to the right lacked 20 per cent while side-flexion to the left lacked 10 per cent. On the fourth and fifth visits transverse oscillatory pressure was repeated as before. During the sixth session, all of the patient's movements were full and pain-free. The pain on her right had also disappeared.

CASE 10. BACK PAIN OF NON-SPINAL ORIGIN

A 33-year-old laborer with pain in his back for no apparent reason went to see his doctor, whose findings were negative. The orthopedic surgeon to whom he was referred also could not pin down the source of the patient's pain, although the radiographical picture indicated slight narrowing of the disc space between L4 and L5. He requested a course of lumbar traction to be tried as an empirical measure.

On examination, all spinal movements were full and pain-free, apart from extension which caused pain at the extreme. Tenderness was present over L1, L3 and L4. The patient reported that his pain was always there, ameliorated only by the pills his doctor had prescribed.

During the first visit, lumbar traction was given for 15 minutes on a friction-free table. There was no change in the patient's symptoms. On the second visit the traction treatment was repeated with indifferent results. The same thing happened during the third and fourth sessions. When the patient arrived for the fifth session he reported that he had suffered severe pain following the last treatment. At the time that he was seen, he was breathing heavily and in great pain. At this point, he was referred back to his doctor with a statement about lack of response to treatment, and a request for this further examination and review.

The doctor, suspecting a respiratory condition, referred the patient to a chest physician who later diagnosed carcinoma of the bronchus after a laboratory report on a bronchial biopsy. This patient died 2 weeks later.

The manipulative therapist sometimes finds himself with a patient who is unsuited for manipulation and who has escaped the screening process which usually takes place before the patient knocks on the manipulative therapist's door. Pain in the back which is the result of reference from a distant pathology occurs frequently in diseases such as gravid impacted uterus, cardiac infarct, pelvic-endometriosis and polycystic kidney disease.

CASE 11. PAIN IN THE BACK RADIATING DOWN THE ANTERIOR ASPECT OF THE RIGHT THIGH

A man of 28 was involved in an automobile accident 3 months prior to his examination. At first he had a dull ache in his lower back and later began to experience pain in the anterior aspect of his right thigh. The dull ache in his back did not bother him as much as the pain in his thigh. The patient was a choreographer and every time he flexed his right knee or extended his right hip, he felt a sharp pain in front of his right thigh. His doctor put him on sick leave and requested that manipulative therapy be tried.

Examination revealed tenderness over L2, L3 and L4 and spasm in these areas on palpation. Lumbar rotation was limited by 50 per cent and 20 per cent to the right and left, respectively. Lumbar rotation to the right caused pain to shoot down the front of the right thigh. Testing of intervertebral joint mobility revealed limitation in L2/L3 and L3/L4 joints. The prone-lying knee-flexion test was positive, causing pain in the right thigh.

Oscillatory rotation with the right leg on top was administered to the lumbar spine. This was done three times, each time for 20 seconds. After treatment there was no significant change in the patient's pain but rotation of the lumbar spine to the right increased by 20 per cent. During the second visit, the patient reported that 4 hours after the last treatment session he had noticed that the pain in his right thigh had diminished. Oscillatory rotation was repeated as before. This oscillatory rotation routine was performed on the third, fourth, fifth and sixth sessions. By the time the patient appeared for the seventh session full lumbar rotational movement in both directions had been restored. The pain reference in his right thigh had also been reduced in intensity and frequency. A specific lumbar rotatory thrust localized to the L3/L4 joint was administered once with the right leg on top. This was followed by complete relief of the dull ache in the back and the pain in the thigh. When the patient was seen for the eighth treatment session, he reported that he had not had any pain since the last treatment. This session ended the treatment program.

CASE 12. PAIN IN THE BACK OF SLOW ONSET

Two weeks prior to examination, a 30-year-old longshoreman felt a "twinge" in his lower back as he lifted a heavy object at work. He did not think much of the pain at the time and it did not stop him from working. On the following working day however, he experienced a dull ache in his back which increased in intensity as he worked. By closing time, his back had become so painful that he was barely able to drive himself home in his car. When he woke up the following morning, he had so much pain in his back that going to work was out of the question. Furthermore, he observed that the pain had spread down to his left buttock and lower limb. His wife called the doctor who confined the patient to bed for a week. It was after this period of confinement that he was referred for treatment.

Examination of the patient revealed that the pain was localized to the lower back with pain reference to the left buttock, the outer side of the thigh down to the outer side of the left leg. The normal lumbar lordosis was reduced with slight deviation of the lumbar spine to the right. Coughing caused pain to shoot down his left leg. The patient found it impossible to side-flex the spine to the left and an attempt to do this evoked spasm in the low back. There was severe limitation of flexion and he tried to flex the lumbar spine by flexing at the hips. Rotation to the left was very limited. The straight-leg-raising test showed 20 degrees and the skin-roll test was positive over L4, L5 and S1.

From the first to the sixth visits, the patient was treated with lumbar traction. Initially the poundage was 35 for 10 minutes on a friction-free table. This was gradually increased to 45 pounds for 20 minutes. On the seventh visit the patient reported that he was considerably better. The pain in his left lower limb had disappeared, and was not located mainly in his lower back and left buttock. He had no more pain when he coughed. Straight-leg-raising was now 60 degrees. Traction was given for 20 minutes with a poundage of 45. On the eighth visit the improvement from previous treatments was maintained but there was no further progress. Oscillatory rotation with the left leg on top was done three times, each time for 20 seconds. On post-treatment assessment, the pain in the back and left buttock was reduced in intensity. During the ninth session the patient was pleased with the progress he had made. He had had no pain since the last visit. However, forward flexion and rotation to the right were both still limited by 15 degrees. Oscillatory rotation as for the last treatment was repeated. Treatment was suspended for 2 weeks and the patient was asked to report back after this period for a reassessment of his condition. He has not been heard from since then.

CASE 13. PAIN IN THE BACK AND RIGHT BUTTOCK OF SUDDEN ONSET

Two days prior to examination a 40-year-old man experienced a sudden pain in his back as he bent down to pick up his morning paper. After this incident he was immobilized for a while. When he finally assumed the upright posture, he realized that he also had pain in his right buttock. He likened the suddenness of the pain to an "explosion" in his back.

On examination, the patient described his back pain as "dull" but his buttock pain as "sharp." Standing exacerbated the buttock pain. There was 50 per cent limitation of side-flexion to the right. Rotation to the right was also limited by 50 per cent. An attempt at extension caused exacerbation of the buttock pain. There was tenderness over L4, L5 and S1 levels.

During the first session oscillatory rotation directed at the lower lumbar spine was administered with the right leg on top. This was done three times, each time for 25 seconds. On post-treatment assessment, the right buttock pain had disappeared but the dull pain in the back was still present. On the second visit, the patient reported that he had no pain in his right buttock and that the dull ache in his back was considerably less. Side-flexion to both sides was full. Rotation to the right was short by 10 per cent. A rotatory thrust was administered, directed first at L4/L5 joint and then to L5/S1. This was followed by complete relief of pain and restoration of full movements.

CASE 14. PAIN IN THE BACK AFTER SPINAL OPERATION

A 42-year-old schoolteacher had a laminectomy to remove the herniated discs between his L4/L5 and L5/S1 joints. This was done 9 months prior to his visit for back pain and the pain reference which he had had in both lower limbs. He had suffered this pain on and off for 5 years prior to the surgery. After the operation, pain in both legs had disappeared and the pain in his back was considerably ameliorated. Two weeks prior to his visit however, the original pain in his back started making its appearance with the same intensity as it had been pre-surgery. The patient, fearing that his old problem might come back, went to see the neurosurgeon who performed the laminectomy. It was he who referred the patient for "gentle manipulation." The surgeon rationalized that the patient's pain was due to post-operative fibrosis in the operation site and that manipulative therapy might help to solve the problem.

When examined, the patient's lumbar movements were short by 50 per cent and all caused pain with the exception of side-flexion to both sides which was full and pain-free. Tenderness was pronounced over L3, L4, L5 and S1. The pain was dull in nature and localized in the lower back and equally bilaterally distributed in relation to the mid-line.

Vertical oscillatory pressure was performed on L3, L4, L5 and S1 levels for 20 seconds on each level, and was repeated two times. On post-treatment assessment, there was a 10 per cent increase in the ranges of movement which had showed limitation, but there was no change in the back pain. The treatment routine was repeated on the second, third and fourth sessions. On the fifth session, the patient reported an improvement in his back pain. He now felt the pain an average of twice a day. At this time, all movements were full with rotation to the right causing slight pain at the extreme. Although the patient was scheduled to attend a sixth session, he did not show up. When contacted later, he was back at work and he thought that he did not need any more treatment.

CASE 15. PAIN IN THE BACK AND LEFT BUTTOCK OF SACROILIAC ORIGIN

When her pregnancy was 6 months in progress, a 25-year-old housewife started having pain in her back and left buttock. At first her pain was ill-defined and made itself felt intermittently after prolonged standing. She suffered through all of this pain, attributing it to part of the inconvenience of pregnancy. In fact, the pain wore off toward the end of her term. However, 3½ months post-partum, the original pain reappeared. Her physician, suspecting a sacroiliac lesion, referred her for manipulative therapy.

Examination revealed that all lumbar movements were full and pain-free with the exception of extension. There was tenderness over the left sacroiliac joint area. Tenderness was detected also in the area of the posterior sacrotuberous ligament on the left. During standing, the iliac crest was raised on the left side and the convexity of the resulting scoliosis was toward the same side. The patient felt relief in a sitting position with her feet elevated higher than the level at which she was sitting.

A rotatory thrust to the left sacroiliac joint was administered. During the treatment, a cracking sound was heard. This maneuver was performed once. After the treatment, the left buttock pain disappeared, leaving a much reduced back pain. During the second session the patient reported that since the last treatment session, she had had pain in her left buttock only once and that had been after washing the dishes at the sink. The pain in her back was also considerably better. Treatment was repeated as for the last time. She was asked to telephone to make an appointment if she had any more problems with her back. She has not been heard from since.

chapter 9

Discussion

At one time or another most adults have had back pain in varying degrees. Yet, despite the fact that backache is as prevalent as the common cold, it has been as puzzling as the Gordian knot and as elusive as the Scarlet Pimpernel! A survey of available literature reveals a pharmacopoeia of solutions none of which can lay claim as the final word in the therapeutic approach toward the well known twinge in the back. This state of affairs only reflects the perplexingly complex entity that is backache.

This chapter will attempt to examine the problematic subject of backache, including its complexities and ramifications. Some questions will also be examined, as well as the attempts which have been made by various authors to answer them. What for instance, is the cause of the common backache? How does manipulation work? What is the role of the physical therapist in the application of manipulative therapy? What are the problems attendant on the teaching of manipulative therapy? How scientific is the chiropractic theory of subluxation?

THE RIDDLE OF BACK PAIN

Most authors who have attempted to examine and explain this multi-faceted problem have directed their attention to one or two facets and have tried to overemphasize certain aspects of the problem. Hackett has directed attention to weak ligaments as the source of back pain.[1] Cyriax' explanation is pressure on nerve roots resulting from disc herniation.[2] Williams' theory has had considerable impact in many quarters.[3] Lumbar lordosis is what he says precipitates backacke. Williams' exercises, designed to correct lumbar lordosis, are a familiar feature in therapeutic regimes designed to alleviate back pain in many physical therapy departments. Mennell's theory of "joint play" and "joint dysfunction" has also enjoyed wide popularity.[4] Schmorl and Junghens, in an attempt to explain back pain, have produced a close description of the late stages of disc pathology.[5] Gray, like Cyriax, believes that the intervertebral disc is the culprit when the cause of back pain is sought.[6] Bourdillon has asked that we look away from the discs when trying to establish the cause of back pain.[7] Charnley has also exculpated the disc and expressed dissatisfaction at the various theories which implicate the intervertebral disc as the primary cause of symptoms.[8] Friberg and Hult made a comparative study of abrodil myelogram and operative findings,[9] and discovered sciatic symptoms in patients who had no disc protrusion. Pedersen and his co-workers have drawn attention to the sinuvertebral nerve fibers as the pain source.[10] Roaf casts doubt on the fact that herniation of a healthy disc occurs.[11] He mentions that disc protrusion is a possible sequel to ischemia following poor nutrition of a disc secondary to infection or trauma.

For many years the diversity of symptoms emanating from spinal joints puzzled the medical profession which did not recognize their source until Mixter and Barr's work partially clarified the problem in 1934.[12] Although much work on the causative factors in backache has been done since then, many gaps in knowledge still exist. There is still some uncertainty as to the type of degeneration which takes place in the intervertebral disc during "cervical spondylosis," for instance.[13] This attractive sounding term was coined by Schmorl in 1927 to describe the long standing degenerative changes in the intervertebral discs producing the symptoms which are familiar to the clinician.[14] This term has enjoyed great favor and often appears on request forms when the physical therapist is consulted for treatment.

One of the interesting conditions which is often encountered in clinical practice is a lesion in any of the upper thoracic intervertebral joints. Such a lesion frequently produces symptoms which mimic the symptoms of a heart condition. A patient who has such a condition ends up with the illusion that his "heart trouble" was cured by manipulation. The chiropractor or manipulator might also share the illusion. The reader might be interested to know that after the injection of hypertonic saline into the left side of the spinous process of the first thoracic spine of subjects, Lewis and Kellgren produced pain in the upper interscapular area and the anterior aspect of the upper chest.[15] Sometimes lesions in the upper thoracic intervertebral joints also simulate Meniere's syndrome, a phenomenon possibly due to the fact that the sympathetic supply to the vessels in the head originates in the first and second thoracic segments, and sometimes in the third thoracic segment. However the mechanism requires investigation.

Attempts to subject manipulative therapy to a thorough scientific investigative process is fraught with difficulties. There are innumerable variables to be considered in order not to confound results, and make findings invalid. Some of the more important of these variables are the problems of diagnosis, the skill of the operator, the total personality profile of the patient and the circumstances in which the treatment is carried out. In addition, backacke has the peculiar characteristic of spontaneous recovery either temporarily or permanently. Attempts to study the effects of manipulation using radiographical investigation have led to conflicting reports. Went and Walter observed that there were no roentgenological changes following manipulation when compared with the anatomical status before treatment.[16] Swezey and Silverman investigated the extent to which displacements in facet joints would go undetected radiographically.[17] They created measured displacements at facet joints of a spinal column from a human skeleton and took standard radiographical views. They observed that vertical displacements which exceeded 4.5 millimeters could be detected, but overriding displacements of 3 millimeters between the fifth and sixth cervical vertebrae and 3.5 millimeters between the fifth lumbar vertebra and the sacrum were not detectable. They suggested that if radiographs were closely scrutinized, facet joint displacements might be more easily detected. This, of course, has implications for manipulative therapy.

One often comes across a grateful patient and a pleased surgeon following a successful laminectomy for the removal of a large herniation. However, it is a well known fact that the long term results of spinal operations for removal of disc protrusions are not as gratifying. It has to be remembered that the purpose of a laminectomy is to relieve pressure on the nerve roots and dural sac. Theoretically, when this is done, the patient should not experience any more pain. Krayenbühl and Zander have analyzed the results of Weber who has made an accurate follow-up study of 459 patients operated on for disc protrusions.[18] Surgery was able to relieve back pain and sciatic symptoms in 40 per cent of the patients. Mennell has pointed out that the partial success or failure of laminectomies might be due to erroneous diagnosis, inadequate post-operative care and the fact that laminectomies do not rectify the mechanical derangement caused by the lesion for which the patient was operated upon.[4]

Spinal fusion has its advocates in some quarters. The rationale for this exercise is that symptoms originate in neighboring synovial joints and spinal fusion ensures that these joints will cease to be the source of pain.

THE PHYSICAL THERAPIST AND MANIPULATION

A great deal of controversy has raged in physical therapy circles regarding whether or not physical therapists should manipulate. The pro-manipulation side seems to be winning the argument, as evidenced by the great enthusiasm displayed by physical therapists at the World Confederation for Physical Therapy held in June, 1974 in Montreal, Canada. When papers on manipulation were read, the conference hall was so packed that many delegates had to stand outside. Mennell has pointed out that the use of manipulative therapy by physical therapists will breathe a new air of "professionalism" into physical therapy,[19] since manipulative therapy will help to get the physical therapist away from the performance of certain non-professional mechanical chores which have earned him the image of a "technician."

For many years in the United Kingdom, it was advocated that manipulative therapy should be included in the syllabus of the Chartered Society of Physiotherapy; but there was no response. Recently however, the subject has been included in the list of post-graduate courses which are organized by that society. Some schools of physiotherapy have added the subject to their normal curricula. The difficulty in teaching the subject to undergraduate physiotherapists has been due to the paucity of teachers with enough expertise in this field.

Questions regarding professional ethics have often been asked regarding the routine use of manipulation by physical therapists. Mennell mentions that in 1969, the Board of Directors of the American Physical Therapy Association (A.P.T.A.) ratified a resolution which had been introduced by the A.P.T.A. House of Delegates.[19] This resolution stated that a physical therapist was free to employ any method or modality of physical therapy known to him for treating a patient referred from a doctor requesting restoration of movement, which is the basic premise of manipulative therapy.

It is a generally accepted opinion that when teaching manipulation to undergraduate physical therapists, the techniques taught should be restricted to the gentler ones similar to the oscillatory techniques described in this book. The more forceful maneuvers should be reserved for post-graduate courses. Students must be taught manipulation not in isolation but in conjunction with the recognition of mechanical lesions, the indications and contraindications of manipulation, and how to vary techniques and actual clinical application.

EDUCATIONAL OPPORTUNITIES AND WORLD ORGANIZATIONS IN MANIPULATIVE THERAPY

The 1960s have seen a gradual expansion of the facilities for teaching manipulative therapy within the medical and physical therapy professions.

The physical therapy curriculum in many schools in Australia and New Zealand includes manipulation. The inauguration of the Manual Therapy Study Group of the Australian Association of New South Wales was seen in 1965. Identical groups have been formed in Australia since then. Mr. G. Maitland and Dr. Burnell have worked hard to establish introductory courses in Adelaide.

In the United States, opportunities to study manipulative therapy are scarce because of the dearth of instructors within the medical or physical therapy professions. To some extent the A.P.T.A. organizes post-graduate courses through the Institute of Orthopedic Physical Therapy of which Mr. S. Paris is the President. This organization, which has now become an arm of the A.P.T.A., is a reformed version of The North American Academy of Manipulation Therapy which was formed in 1967 to promote manipulative therapy. Its conversion to the Institute of Orthopedic Physical Therapy took place in 1974. Most of the opportunities to learn about the subject still exist within the osteopathic and chiropractic professions.

In the United Kingdom, most of the opportunities for education in manipulative therapy are in the hands of the osteopathic profession. In the later part of the 1920s and 1930s some medical practitioners went to the United States and took post-graduate courses in osteopathic colleges. It was they who originated the London College of Osteopathy in 1945. This college provides post-graduate training for doctors who are interested in osteopathy. The British School of Osteopathy, also located in London, has a 4-year program for non-medical students. The graduates of this program refrain from giving advice on medical matters and confine their treatments to the locomotor system, in contrast to their American counterparts who have full legal medical status.

The year 1963 saw the inauguration of the British Association of Manipulative Medicine. In 1965 the first Congress of the International Federation of Manual Medicine was held in London. The North American Academy of Manipulative Medicine was inaugurated in San Francisco in 1964. The International Association of Manual Therapy, made up of 25 member-nations, was formed at about the same time, with the British Association of Manipulative Medicine as its first member. The year 1971 witnessed the formation of the Australian Association of Manipulative Medicine.

SCIENCE VERSUS CHIROPRACTIC PHILOSOPHY

Opinion about chiropractors is split down the middle, some people swearing by them and others considering them a menace in the arena of health care. The favorable opinion which chiropractors enjoy in some quarters obviously reflects the pleasant experience these people have had with them.

One of the main reasons for the antagonism of the medical profession toward chiropractic is that it has not been able to demonstrate scientifically the validity of chiropractic's theory of subluxation as the basis of disease causation. The implication of this theory is that subluxation causes a disturbance of the distribution of nervous flow.[20–22] It is a general assumption among members of the medical profession that if the chiropractic concept of disease causation receives their approbation, the very foundation of scientific medicine which has evolved over the centuries will be questionable.

The public relations organs of the two chiropractic associations in the United States, including their lobbying and advertisement machinery, are very impressive. Chiropractic gives the impression to the public and the policymakers in government that they are a persecuted profession and are not to blame for the vendetta between them and the medical profession. They also plug the theme that interprofessional quarreling is uncalled for since there is much room for all health professions to co-exist peacefully.[23]

E. S. Crelin has done some important work aimed at investigating the validity of the chiropractic theory of subluxation.[24] At the time of writing, Crelin was a Professor of Anatomy and Chairman of the Human Growth and Development Study at Yale University School of Medicine,

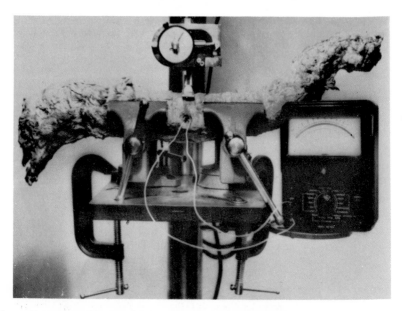

FIG. 9.1. Adult vertebral column, in Crelin's experiment, held by two vises on a drill press platform. A wire from a V.O.M. meter is wrapped around the 10th thoracic spinal nerve. The other wire has been placed on the side of the intervertebral foramen.

Reproduced from Am. Sci., *61:* (No. 5, Sept.–Oct.), 577, 1973. By permission of the Editor.

New Haven, Connecticut. He has published over 100 papers on the development, structure and physiology of bones and joints and he is a well known authority in these fields. The rest of the chapter will be devoted to his investigation of the chiropractic concept.

Crelin studied the effects of applying stresses on the cadaverous vertebral columns of 6 individuals: 3 were infants—2 males and 1 female; the remainder were adults—also 2 males and 1 female. The specific purpose of the study was to investigate whether there was interference with nerve transmission resulting from deviation of the body segments of the spine from their normal juxtaposition. Chiropractors have never subjected the spine to an experimental situation to determine how much vertebral displacement would be needed before a spinal nerve was compromised at the intervertebral foramen, precipitating a pathological status.

Metal vises were clamped to the platform of a drill press to give support to the experimental spine while a compressive force was applied (Figure 9.1). Crelin found that after applying 200 pounds to the adult spine, the relationship of the spinal nerve to its intervertebral foramen remained

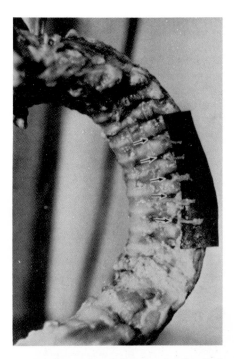

FIG. 9.2. Application of maximal flexion in Crelin's experiment. The compressive force entered on this spinal column of a newborn is made by the pressure foot of a drill press. A black piece of paper has been placed behind the fifth to ninth left thoracic spinal nerves. *Arrows* point to the intervertebral foramina.

Reproduced from Am. Sci., *61:* (No. 5, Sept.–Oct.), 580, 1973. By permission of the Editor.

unchanged. He even applied 1000 pounds to one of the vertebrae. Even though this caused a collapse of the vertebral body, the relationship of the nerve to its intervertebral foramen remained the same. After applying maximal compressive force to the spines of the infants, there were still areas of space between the spinal nerves and their intervertebral foramina. When the spines of the adults and infants were maximally twisted, flexed (Figure 9.2) in the forward direction and side-flexed, the spinal nerves did not show any significant sign of pressure.

Crelin's study showed experimentally that the chiropractic theory of subluxation could not be justified.

REFERENCES

1. Hackett, J. S. *Joint Ligament Relaxation*. Charles C Thomas, Springfield, Illinois, 1957.
2. Cyriax, J. *Textbook of Orthopaedic Medicine*, vol. I. Cassell, London, 1962.
3. Williams, P. C. *The Lumbosacral Spine*. McGraw-Hill, New York, 1965.
4. Mennell, J. *Back Pain*. Little Brown, Boston, 1960.
5. Schmorl, G. and Junghens, H. *The Human Spine in Health and Disease*. Grune and Stratton, New York, 1959.
6. Gray, F. J. The lumbar disc syndrome. A preliminary report on a method of treatment combining body weight, traction on an inclined plane and manipulation. Med. J. Aust., *1:* 958–961, 1967.
7. Bourdillon, J. *Spinal Manipulation*. Heinemann, London, 1970.
8. Charnley, J. Physical change in the prolapsed disc. Lancet, *2:* 43–44, 1958.
9. Friberg, S. and Hult, L. Comparative study of abrodil myelogram and operative findings. Acta Orthopaedic. Scand., *20:* 303–314, 1951.
10. Pedersen, H. E., Blunck, C. F. T. and Gardiner, E. Anatomy of the lumbosacral posterior rami. J. Bone Joint Surg., *38A:* 377–391, 1956.
11. Roaf, R. Physical changes in the prolapsed discs. Lancet, *2:* 265–266, 1958.
12. Mixter, W. J. and Barr, J. S. Rupture of the intervertebral disc with involvement of the spinal canal. N. Engl. J. Med., *211:* 210–215, 1934.
13. Perkins, G. *Orthopaedics*. University of London Althone Press, London, 1961.
14. Schmorl, G. Deutsch Ortho. Casellreh, *21:* 3, 1927.
15. Lewis, T. and Kellgren, J. H. Observations relating to referred pain. Clin. Sci., *4:* 47–71, 1939.
16. Went, H. and Walter, R. The effect of manipulative treatment of the spinal column (Zum wirkungsmecharismus der chiropractic). Arch. Orthop. Unfall-Chir., *49:* 480–485, 1958.
17. Swezey, R. L. and Silverman, J. R. Radiographic demonstration of induced vertebral facet displacements. Arch. Phys. Med. Rehabil., 244–249, 1971.
18. Krayenbühl, H. and Zander, E. *Documenta Geigy. Acta Rheumatologica. Herniation of Lumbar and Cervical Intervertebral Discs*, No. 1, J. R. Geigy, Basel, Switzerland, 1956.
19. Mennell, J. The rationale of manipulation. Phys. Ther., *50:* 2, 1970.
20. Data Sheet on Chiropractic. Department of Investigation, American Medical Association, Chicago, 1970.
21. *International Chiropractic Review*. International Chiropractic Association, March, 1964.
22. Smith, R. L. *At Your Risk. The Case Against Chiropractic*. Pocket Books, New York, 1969.
23. Maloney, R. Letter to Editor (Chiropractic). Phys. Ther., *53:* 1217–1218, 1973.
24. Crelin, E. S. A scientific test of the chiropractic theory. Am. Sci., *61:* 573–580, 1974.

chapter 10 Conclusion

This book constitutes a modest attempt at examining the subject of manipulation of the spine concisely, yet comprehensively, using physical signs and symptoms as guides for treatment. The author has permitted cold light to play on the facets of the situation and no dark corners have been spared. The obligation rests on the reader to view the subject through unprejudiced eyes and to make up his mind about the merits and demerits of the subject. It is a subject which has witnessed much controversy and heated debates among those whose honest wish is to relieve the agonies of the ubiquitous back pain—a frequent portender and co-rider of incapacity, suffering and economic loss in the community.

The huge economic toll which back pain takes on communities is unquestionable. Hayes notes that the sum of 40 million dollars is spent on the medical and surgical care of back pain in the state of Michigan.[1] Great Britain loses 5 million days a year due to back pain among workers.[2] The recognition of this economic drain prompted the formation of a back pain research association.

Manipulation as a therapeutic modality has languished in the doldrums of oblivion and neglect for too long. Even in some quarters of medicine, potential critics have sealed their lips, for fear that their scurrilous statements about the subject might give it negative recognition!

The efficacy of manipulation for dealing with back pain has been noted by some authors. Pringle mentions that the time which workers took off because of back pain was reduced by 50 per cent after the introduction of manipulative therapy.[3] Chrisman and his co-workers report that 20 out of 29 patients who presented signs of ruptured intervertebral discs had "good" or "excellent" results after treatment with manipulative therapy.[4] These patients had been subjected to traditional conventional approaches without success. Cyriax refers to the work of Myrian who made comparisons between the results obtained by conventional methods and manipulation.[5] Four per cent of the patients treated by conventional methods were "well" as compared to 23.4 per cent treated by manipulation. Twenty-six per cent of the patients whereas treated by conventional methods were unable to return to work, whereas all of the patients treated by manipulation were able to return to work. Thiery-Mieg reports excellent results of treatment by manipulation of the cervical spine in nine cases of trigeminal neuralgia.[6] Hirschfield states that results from manipulative therapy are superior to traditional conservative methods.[7]

The time has come for manipulative therapy to be given pride of place among the various modalities for relieving human pain. Wilson has made a plea to consultants in orthopedics and physical medicine to accept manipulation more widely and to participate in the training of doctors on the subject.[8] Barbor mentions that manipulative therapy should become an everyday treatment.[9] When the use of manipulative therapy is advocated however, its limitations should also be recognized. It is not a panacea as some exponents would have us believe. On the other hand it is a modality which possesses more potential than is realized, especially in the medical community. Many medically disillusioned patients who had sought relief in vain in the doctors' offices or hospitals have gotten rid of their pain through the hands of lay manipulators, osteopaths or chiropractors.

Attention is usually drawn away from the efficacy of manipulation by mentioning its dangers. No surgeon has stopped operating on patients because of the potentially dangerous situation of surgery. People have not condemned surgery because an occasional patient has died under anesthesia or suffered a fatal hemorrhage. By the same token, it would not be fair to condemn manipulation because of the previous occasions in which patients have been made worse. Usually it is the manipulator who should be indicted, not manipulation. With a sound background in anatomy, meticulous examination, pre- and post-treatment assessment and sensitivity to contraindications, it is almost impossible to hurt the patient. Accidents are a rarity when the correct technique is performed well for the appropriate conditions. The doctor's diagnostic accuracy is also very helpful. The results of a manipulative maneuver reflect the expertise of the operator. The integration of psychomotor and cognitive skills in achieving an accurate adjustment is the hallmark of a good manipulative therapist.

Some of the supporters and critics of manipulation often refer to the subject as "unorthodox." The patient who appears in the treatment room with back pain wants something done to relieve his pain. He is not interested and invariably cannot understand the doctrinal arguments and what the quarrel is all about. Does it really matter how pain is relieved? Arguing about the method employed is a mere academic exercise which does not help the situation. An "orthodox" method which does not relieve the patient's pain is of no use to him.

Traditional methods of treating back pain in the form of heat, massage and exercises still have their place but in many instances they bear the tinge of an anachronistic approach. In many cases they stand as relics of the days when back pain was believed to have a muscular basis. Since attention has been shifted to articular lesions as the basis of back pain, it stands to reason that treatment should be directed at the offending joint.

In closing this book it would be appropriate to quote a statement from the writing of the illustrious British surgeon, Sir Robert Jones.[10]

We should mend our ways rather than abuse the unqualified. Dramatic successes at their hands should cause us to enquire as to the reasons. It is not wise or dignified to waste time denouncing their many mistakes for we cannot hide the fact that their successes are our failures.

This statement which is over 40 years old is still very relevant today.

REFERENCES

1. Hayes, C. F. *Neckache and Backache* (Gurdjian and Thomas, C. M., Eds.) Charles C Thomas, Springfield, Illinois, 1970.
2. Cyriax, J. The pros and cons of manipulation. Lancet, *7333:* 571–573, 1964.
3. Pringle, B. Approach to intervertebral disc lesions. Trans. Assoc. Indus. Med. Off., *5:* 127, 1956.
4. Chrisman, O. D., Mittnacht, A. and Snook, G. A. A study of the results following rotatory manipulation in the lumbar intervertebral disc syndrome. J. Bone Joint Surg., *46A:* 517–524, 1964.
5. Cyriax, J. *Textbook of Orthopaedic Medicine,* vol. II. Williams & Wilkins, Baltimore, 1969.
6. Thiery-Mieg, J. Treatment by manipulation in facial neuralgia (Intérêt de la physiothérapie manipulative dans les algies faciales). Ann. Med. Phys., *11:* 52–56, 1959.
7. Hirschfield, P. F. Die konservative Behandlung de lumbalen Bandscheibenvor falls nach der methode Cyriax. Deutsch. Med. Wschr., *87:* 299–304, 1962.
8. Wilson, D. G. Manipulative treatment in general practice. Lancet, *7237:* 1013–1015, 1962.
9. Barbor, R. C. Rationale of manipulation of joints. Arch. Phys. Med., *43:* 615–620, 1962.
10. Jones, R. Manipulation as a therapeutic measure. Proc. R. Soc. Med., *25:* 1405, 1932.

Index

Anatomy, 12–22
  cutaneous innervation, scheme, 31–32
  joints of vertebral column, 17–18
  muscles of extremities, innervation, 34–35
  spinal column, 12–22
  vertebrae, 13–17
Apophyseal joints (see Joints)
Arm pain and paresthesia associated with neck pain, case history, 98–99
Atlanto-axial joints (see Joints)
Atlanto-occipital joints (see Joints)

Back pain (see also Pain)
  case histories, 101–102, 104–108
    and pain in left buttock, of sacroiliac origin, 107–108
    and pain in right buttock, of sudden onset, 106–107
    of non-spinal origin, 104
    of slow onset, 105–106
    radiating to thigh, 105
  diagnosis (see Examination of patient)
  economic toll, 117
  riddle of, discussion, 109–111
  traditional therapy and manipulative therapy, comparative efficacy, 118–119
Bonesetting
  Hood's contributions, 5
  in history of manipulative therapy, 5
  Paget's contributions, 5
Buttocks, pain associated with back pain, case histories, 106–108

Case histories, 96–108
Cervical headache (see Headache, cervical)
Cervical region (see also Neck)
  flexion, examination of, 39–40
  locking technique, 56
  manipulative techniques, 51–56
  oscillatory pressure
    transverse, 52–53
    vertical, 51–52
  oscillatory rotation, 53–54
  oscillatory techniques, clinical application, 72
  rotatory thrust, 53–54
  traction (see Traction, cervical)
Chest and shoulder pain, case history, 102–103
Chiropractic
  current status, 8, 113–116
  history, 6
  "mixers," philosophy of, 6

Palmer's contributions, 6
philosophical schools, 6
radiologic examination, 8
"straights," philosophy of, 6
subluxation philosophy, 6
  experimental investigations, 114–116
  techniques, as components of manipulative therapy, 47–48
Clinical application of spinal manipulation (see also Manipulative therapy; Techniques; and the specific condition or anatomic site), 67–81
  case histories, 96–108
  dangers and contraindications, 78–80
  duration and frequency of treatment, 76–77
  manipulative thrusts, 73–74
  operator/patient relationship, 77–78
  oscillatory techniques, 69–73
  postmanipulative reactions, 74–75
  recording of treatments, 77
  successful manipulation, prerequisites, 80
  traction, 84
  vacuum snaps, explanation and implications, 74
Compression tests
  sacroiliac joints
    horizontal, 42
    vertical, 42–43
  spinous processes, vertical, 43
Contraindications
  of manipulative therapy, 78–79
  of traction, 94–95
Costovertebral joints (see Joints)
Crelin's experiments, in investigation of subluxation theory, 114–116
Cutaneous innervation, anatomy, 31–32
Cyriax, James
  contributions
    to disc philosophy, 9
    to manipulative therapy, 9
  techniques
    as components of manipulative therapy, 9, 47
    in nonspecific manipulations, 49

Diagnosis (see Examination of Patient)
Discs (see Intervertebral discs)

Effleurage, clinical application, 75
Ely's test (prone-lying knee-flexion), 36
End-feel test, 43
Examination of patient, 23–45
  cervical flexion, 39–40
  cutaneous innervation, anatomy, 31–32

Ely's test, 36
end-feel test, 43
flexion, 37, 39–41
general considerations, 43–45
gross spinal movements, 36–38
hip-rolling test, 45
history, 26–29
horizontal compression test, sacroiliac joints, 42
initial questioning and observation, 25–26
intervertebral mobility tests, 38
Lasègue's test, 37
localization of pain, 30–33
lumbar flexion, 40–41
muscle weakness, 33
muscular innervation of extremities, anatomy, 34–35
neck movements, side-flexion, 37
neurological, 33–36
objectives, 24–25
occipito-atlantal movement, 38–39
paresis, 33
pressure-on-the-head test, for determining value of cervical traction, 85
radiologist's report, 45
reflexes, 33
sacroiliac joints, compression tests, 42–43
sensory changes, 33
skin-rolling test, 44
spinous processes, vertical compression test, 43
straight-leg-raising test, 37
thoracic resilience, 43–44
thoracic rotation, 40–41
traction test, for determining value of cervical traction, 85
vertical compression test
sacroiliac joints, 42–43
spinous processes, 43
Extremities
muscular innervation, anatomy, 34–35
pain and paresthesia of arm with neck pain, case history, 98–99
pain in thigh radiating from back pain, case history, 105

Facet apposition locking, technique, 49
Facet joints (see Joints)
Flexion tests (see Examination of patient)

Galen, contributions to manipulative therapy, 5
Gibbus, traction for (historical), 83
Girdle pain around trunk, case history, 103–104

Headache
cervical
case history, 96–97

origin and manipulative treatment, 75–76
oscillatory pressure for, 76
osteopathic therapy (historical), 7
Hippocrates, contributions to manipulative therapy, 4
Hip-rolling test, 45
Hood, Wharton, contributions in bonesetting, 5
Horizontal compression test (see Compression tests)

Intervertebral discs
anatomy, 19
herniated, lumbar traction for, 94
in back pain, concepts of, 9
lesions, Cyriax' concepts, 9
Intervertebral mobility tests, 38

Joints
apophyseal, anatomy, 17
atlanto-axial
anatomy, 17
manipulation techniques, 55
atlanto-occipital (occipito-atlantal)
anatomy, 17
manipulation techniques, 54
movement, examination of, 38–39
costovertebral, anatomy, 17
dysfunction, and disease, theory, 8
facet, anatomy, 17
facet apposition locking, technique, 49
manipulation, history of, 8
play of, and disease, theory, 8
sacroiliac
anatomy, 18
counterclockwise rotation, technique, 65–66
examination, 42
horizontal compression test, 42
rotatory thrust, technique, 65
vertical compression test, 42–43
vertical thrust, technique, 64
vertebral column, anatomy, 17–18
zygapophyseal, anatomy, 17

Kaltenborn's contributions to manipulative therapy, 10
Knee-flexion test (see Ely's test)
Kyphosis, in diagnosis of back pain, 25

Lasègue's test (straight-leg-raising test), 36
Leverage of movement, technique, 49
Ligaments of spinal column, anatomy, 18–19
Locking technique
in cervical manipulation, 56
facet apposition, 49
Lordosis, in diagnosis of back pain, 25–29

Lumbar region
  flexion, examination of, 40–41
  manipulative techniques, 60–64
    oscillatory, clinical application, 73
    oscillatory pressure, vertical, 57
    oscillatory rotation, 60–61
    "pump-handle" technique, 62–63
    rotation, 62–64
    specific rotation, 63–64
    vertical thrust, 61–62
  traction (see Traction, lumbar)

Maigne, Robert, concepts of, 9
Maitland, G. D.
  contributions to vertebral manipulation, 10, 11
  oscillatory techniques, 50
Manipulation (see Manipulative therapy)
Manipulative therapy
  case histories, 96–108
  chiropractic and (see Chiropractic)
  clinical applications (see also Clinical applications), 67–81
  contraindications, 78–79
  current status, 8–11, 118–119
  Cyriax' contributions and methods, 9, 47, 49
  dangers, as compared to other disciplines, 3
  definition, 2–3
  education for, 2, 112–113
  history, 4–11
  incidence, in current practice, 3
  Kaltenborn's contributions, 10
  Maigne's concepts, 9
  Maitland's contributions, 10, 11, 50
  Mennell philosophy and techniques, 8, 47
  misconceptions, 2–3
  mobilization and manipulation, concepts, 9, 11
  osteopathy and (see Osteopathy)
  painlessness and opposite motion, concept of, 9
  physical therapist's role, 112–113
  schools of thought, 4–11
  selection of, 24–25, 68–69
  techniques (see Techniques)
  world organizations, 112–113
Manipulative thrusts (see Thrusts)
Mechanics of spinal column, 12–22
Mennell's contributions to joint manipulation, 8
Mennell's techniques, as components of manipulative therapy, 47
"Mixers," chiropractic philosophy, 6
Mobilization and manipulation
  Maigne's concepts, 9
  Maitland's concepts, 11
Movement

  leverage, technique, 49
  types of, in spinal column, 19–21
Muscles
  of extremities, innervation, 34–35
  weakness, examination for, 33

Neck (see also Cervical region)
  side-flexion movements, examination of, 37
Neck pain, case histories
  dull, at back of neck, 98
  severe, of sudden onset, 97–98
  whiplash injury, 99–100
  with pain and paresthesia in both arms, 98–99
Neurological examination, 33–36

Occipito-atlantal joints (see Joints)
Oscillatory pressure
  cervical region, 51–55
    transverse, 52–53
    vertical, 51–52
  for cervical headache, 76
  lumbar spine, vertical, 57
  thoracic region
    transverse, 57–58
    vertical, 56–57
Oscillatory rotation
  cervical region, 53–54
  lumbar region, 60–61
Oscillatory techniques, 49–50
  clinical application, 69–73
Osteopathy
  current status, 7–8
  definition, 7
  history, 6–8
  philosophy, 6–8
  Still's contributions, 6–7
  techniques, as components of manipulative therapy, 47

Paget, James, contributions to bonesetting, 5
Pain (see also Back pain; Neck pain)
  case histories, 96–108
  diagnosis, 23–45
  localization, 30–33
Painlessness and opposite motion, concept of, 9
Palmer, Daniel David, contributions to chiropractic, 6
Paresis, examination for, 33
Paresthesia and pain of both arms, associated with neck pain, case history, 98–99
Pettrisage, clinical application, 75
Physical therapist's role in manipulative therapy, 112–113
Prone-lying knee-flexion test (Ely's test), 36

"Pump-handle" technique, for lumbar rotation, 62–63

Radiologic examination, by chiropractors, 8
Radiologist's report, significance of, in initial examination, 45
Reflexes, tests of, 33
Rotation
counterclockwise, of sacroiliac joint, technique, 65–66
lumbar, techniques, 62–64
oscillatory (see Oscillatory rotation)
thoracic, examination of, 40–41
Rotatory thrust (see Thrusts)

Sacroiliac joint (see Joints)
Scapular region, "stabbing" pain, case history, 100–101
Scoliosis, in diagnosis of back pain, 25–29
Sensory changes, examination for, 33
Shoulder and chest pain, case history, 102–103
Skin-rolling test, 45
Spinal column
anatomy, 12–22
mechanics, 12–22
movements, 19–21
gross, examination of, 36–38
Spinal manipulation (see Manipulative therapy, also Techniques)
Spinal traction (see Traction)
Spinous processes
surface anatomy, 21
vertical compression test, 43
Still, Andrew Taylor, contributions to osteopathy, 6–7
Straight-leg-raising test (Lasègue's test), 36
"Straights," chiropractic philosophy, 6
Subluxation
chiropractic philosophy, 6
experimental investigations, 114–116

Techniques of spinal manipulation (see also Manipulative therapy, and the specific procedure or site), 47–66
atlanto-axial manipulation, 55
cervical region, 51–56
chiropractic components, 47–48
clinical application (see Clinical application)
counterclockwise rotation, sacroiliac joint, 65–66
direct manipulations, 48
facet apposition locking, 49
indirect manipulations, 48
leverage of movement, 49
locking technique, 49, 56
lumbar region, 57, 60–64

manipulative thrust, 50–51
Non-specific manipulations, 49
occipito-atlantal manipulation, 54
oscillatory pressure, cervical region
transverse, 52–53
vertical, 51–52
oscillatory pressure, thoracic region
transverse, 57–58
vertical, 56–57
oscillatory rotation
cervical region, 53–54
lumbar region, 60–61
oscillatory techniques, 49–50
clinical application, 69–73
osteopathic components, 47–48
positioning of area of spine under treatment, 48–49
"pump-handle" technique, for lumbar rotation, 62–63
rotation, lumbar, 62–64
rotatory thrust
cervical, 53–54
sacroiliac, 65
sacroiliac joint, 64–66
selection of, 24–25, 68–69
specific manipulations, 48
specific rotation, lumbar, 63–64
thoracic region, 56–60
lower, 59–60
middle, 59–60
upper, 58–59
traction (see Traction)
vertical thrust
lumbar region, 61–62
mid- and lower thoracic, 59–60
sacroiliac joint, 64
Tests (see Examination of patient)
Thigh pain, radiating from back pain, case history, 105
Thoracic region
manipulative techniques, 56–60
oscillatory pressure
transverse, 57–58
vertical, 56–57
oscillatory techniques, clinical application, 72
vertical thrust, 59–60
Thoracic resilience, test of, 43–44
Thoracic rotation, examination of, 40–41
Thrusts
manipulative
clinical application, 73–74
technique, 50–51
rotatory
cervical, 53–54
sacroiliac joint, 65
vertical
lumbar, 61–62
sacroiliac joint, 64
thoracic, 59–60

Traction, 82–95
  continuous, 83
  contraindications, 94–95
  definition, 82–83
  for a gibbus, historical, 83
  history, 82–83
  indications for, 84
  intermittent, 83
  methods, 83–84
  rhythmic, 84
  sustained, 83
Traction, cervical
  contraindications, 90
  electronic machine for, 89
  overhead traction unit for, 88
  pressure-on-the-head test, 85
  techniques
    horizontal, 85–87
    in a sitting position, 87–89
    in a standing position, 89–92
    intermittent sustained, 87–88
  traction test, 85
Traction, lumbar
  equipment for, 91–94
  indications and contraindications, 94

  intermittent, efficacy of, 94
  sustained, efficacy of, 94
  techniques, 91–94
Transverse oscillatory pressure (see Oscil-
    latory pressure)
Trauma
  in diagnosis of back pain, 28–30
  resulting from manipulative therapy,
    78–79
Trunk, girdle pain, case history, 103–104

Vacuum snaps, definition and implica-
    tions, 74
Vertebrae, anatomy, 13–17
Vertical compression test (see Compres-
    sion tests)
Vertical oscillatory pressure (see Oscilla-
    tory pressure)
Vertical thrust (see Thrusts)

Whiplash injury, case history, 99–100

X-ray examination (see Radiology)

Zygapophyseal joints (see Joints)